To José
In appreciation
of who you
are, and
your caring
ways
Joan

AF850750

Women as Healers, Women as Patients

To the memory of Julia de Burgos (1917–1953),
a woman for our time

YO MISMA FUI MI RUTA

Yo quise ser como los hombres quisieron que yo fuese:
un intento de vida.
Un juego al escondite con mi ser.
Pero yo estaba hecha de presentes,
y mis pies planos sobre la tierra promisora
no resistían caminar hacia atrís,
y seguían adelante, adelante,
burlando las cenizas para alcanzar el beso
de los senderos nuevos.

I MYSELF WAS MY ROAD

I wanted to be what men wanted me to be:
an attempt at life.
A game of hide and seek with myself.
But I was already formed,
and my feet flat upon the promised land
could not endure walking backwards,
and kept going forwards, forwards,
mocking the ashes in order to reach the kiss
of new ways.

Women as Healers, Women as Patients

Mental Health Care and Traditional Healing in Puerto Rico

Joan Koss-Chioino

UNIV DUNELM

Westview Press
BOULDER • SAN FRANCISCO • OXFORD

23 MAR 2011

3080468

Cover illustration and poems in Spanish on pp. iii and 90 reprinted from Julia de Burgos, Cuadernos de Poesia *(San Juan, Puerto Rico: Instituto de Cultura Puertorriqueña, 1964). Poems used by permission of the Instituto de Cultura Puertorriqueña; cover illustration used by permission of the Instituto and Torres Martinó. English translations of poems by Joan Koss-Chioino.*

This Westview softcover edition is printed on acid-free paper and bound in library-quality, coated covers that carry the highest rating of the National Association of State Textbook Administrators, in consultation with the Association of American Publishers and the Book Manufacturers' Institute.

All rights reserved. No part of this publication may be reproduced or transmitted in any form or by any means, electronic or mechanical, including photocopy, recording, or any information storage and retrieval system, without permission in writing from the publisher.

Copyright © 1992 by Westview Press, Inc.

Published in 1992 in the United States of America by Westview Press, Inc., 5500 Central Avenue, Boulder, Colorado 80301-2877, and in the United Kingdom by Westview Press, 36 Lonsdale Road, Summertown, Oxford OX2 7EW

Library of Congress Cataloging-in-Publication Data
Koss-Chioino, Joan.
Women as healers, women as patients : mental health care and traditional healing in Puerto Rico / by Joan Koss-Chioino.
p. cm.
Includes bibliographical references.
ISBN 0-8133-8321-8
1. Women—Mental health services—Puerto Rico. 2. Women healers—Puerto Rico. 3. Folk medicine—Puerto Rico. I. Title.
RC451.4.W6K67 1992
362.2'082—dc20 91-16538
CIP

362.2082097295
KOS

Printed and bound in the United States of America

The paper used in this publication meets the requirements of the American National Standard for Permanence of Paper for Printed Library Materials Z39.48-1984.

10 9 8 7 6 5 4 3 2 1

In memory of Pete (A. I. Hallowell)
and for all my sisters in feeling,
Jean S., Libbet C., Fredeswinda R.,
Helga U., and Mili L.

Contents

Foreword

He still took his brother's frivolous activities as a personal affront. . . . But he no longer tried to drag him to the hospital to make him look at suffering up close, hoping against hope that the pain of others might move his bird-of-passage heart.

—Isabel Allende, *The House of the Spirits*

This book on women as healers and patients in Puerto Rico is a very different kind of ethnography. Its subject matter follows the established scholarly traditions of medical anthropology; at the same time, it offers unique clinical insights to therapists in mental health occupations. Joan Koss-Chioino provides us with an insider's perspective on Puerto Rican Spiritism through narratives concerning healing from spirit mediums, other healers, and patients. Her accounts are personal and reveal the inner emotional conflicts and concerns of those touched by spirits. Koss-Chioino herself experienced the emotional depths that an initiation into mediumship entails. At the same time, as an anthropologist and skilled psychotherapist, she is able to observe and give meaning to those experiences.

Koss-Chioino therefore achieves a kind of integration of the emic and the etic that makes this study truly unique. For her integration is primarily a result not of comparing cognitive explanatory models of illness and disease or of analyzing symbolic systems but of capturing the emotional conflicts of real people, how they are persuaded, and how they are compelled to discover the spiritual forces in their lives. Koss-Chioino's integration comes from the heart.

Spiritism in Puerto Rico is a healing process that offers an explanation for illness and for other problems in life. It is also a way to understand human relationships in the world in general and, as such, is a cosmological system shared by participants. Healing therefore is a process of religious conversion, consisting of experientially verifying and reaffirming the truths of the system.

Koss-Chioino used well her background as a psychotherapist to develop the Therapist-Spiritist Project that is the subject of this book. The Project demonstrates how traditional healing systems and healers might be brought into congenial liaison with the biomedical system, thus rendering a more holistic treatment of patients. Koss-Chioino discovers that seemingly different, even antagonistic, healing systems such as biomedicine and Spiritism have many elements in common when their metaphors of human experience are translated into the terms of the other. She shows, furthermore, how the personal forces in the lives of women Spiritist healers, mental health professionals, and doctors in mental health clinics in Puerto Rico have much in common. This book therefore should prove to be of great value to clinicians and clinical administrators in settings in the United States and abroad where alternative healing systems coexist in the communities they serve.

Koss-Chioino documents medical doctors' and mental health workers' claims that their own life traumas produced the motivation for pursuing their healing science and art. Their stories are compared to those of the Spiritist healers who are invited into the clinics to explore a collaboration with the mental health system. Koss-Chioino discovers that the women in this more socially underprivileged group were drawn to the art of traditional healing by their own suffering and in that way shared a developmental path somewhat in common with their more formally educated sisters.

From a psychoanalytic perspective, Koss-Chioino's medical healers and traditional folk healers are alike in that they respond to the traumatic events of their lives by developing defense mechanisms of overcompensation: mastering the trauma by turning their passivity into activity, using intellectualization, and exhibiting reaction-formation. Such defenses represent the ego's adaptive capabilities and protect the individual from experiencing painful affects associated with developmental traumas. Egotism and arrogance are traits that do not often survive devastating life traumas. Such events are more likely to humiliate and humble their victims, resulting in a humility that makes these people more approachable than they might otherwise have been.

Healers with motivations born of their own experiences of suffering often have a quality of conviction about their calling. This seems to be true across cultures, as Eliade has discussed in his portrayal of shamanism.[1] My own studies of Inuit shamanism tell much the same story. Shamans-to-be often have an affliction or peculiarity in childhood. Commonly, they are orphans. Experienced healers, seeing in the neophytes a particular sensitivity, invite them to learn the shamanistic arts. Others are called to shamanism by their guardian spirits. In either case, shamanistic initiation is accomplished by means of an emotionally charged experience by which one becomes acquainted with spiritual forces. In our own society, such paradigms are reified as the "psyche" and are understood as psychological forces that conflict with one another and with the self (as do spirits). Neophyte shamans must also be brought to a state of self-knowledge by means of a series of painful regressions whereby they dissect themselves and reassemble themselves bone by bone and muscle by muscle into better, sturdier beings. Shamans are often transvestite and bisexual—forging the male and female aspects of their inner selves into one. Only by going through such a personal breakdown and subsequently being restored can one become a shaman and healer. Those who are thought by others to have endured less are unconvincing as shamans and are considered false.

So too in our own society, we sometimes encounter young doctors who are not yet true healers—medical students and residents who have not experienced enough human suffering and therefore do not radiate the empathetic understanding required to heal others. Their motivations to become physicians may develop from sources other than their own experiences of suffering: perhaps from a fascination with technology and its power to manipulate and do things for and to people or from traumas unresolved and too deeply buried in the past of their own lives to be available for identification with the suffering of others. We trust, however, that during their internship and residency they will eventually be exposed to, and identify with, their patients' suffering and thereby become more sensitive.

Koss-Chioino focuses her project on women as healers, which offers a novel perspective. That it is so novel is perhaps a reflection of the role of women in society having been not only unheralded but also unexamined. Women have suffered from this neglect and from many other aspects of their traditionally underprivileged and exploited status vis-à-vis males in our own as well as in Puerto Rican society. As Koss-Chioino documents, it is perhaps because of the suffering associated with women's role in society that women obtain a natural calling to healing. Of course, males suffer too because of many other kinds of vicissitudes in their own lives. But, unlike women, men in Puerto Rico are not socialized to acknowledge their failings or weaknesses to others, or even to themselves, and for this and other reasons are less likely to become healers.

Going through illness or trauma, and realizing and acknowledging those experiences, provides healers, whether biomedically orthodox or traditional, with unique coping options to offer to patients. Patients often have natural confidence in such healers and are inclined to return to them to seek their counsel. The bonds of mutual struggle are often immediate and strong—a factor in the effectiveness of self-help groups such as Alcoholics Anonymous and Alliance for the Mentally Ill.

Koss-Chioino reveals a complementarity, a circular puzzle, uniting healers and patients. Illness or disorder breaks people down; they reintegrate and compensate for their problems by becoming healers themselves. Their personal experiences provide their own motivation as well as a natural empathic bond to patients, who in turn seek someone with such sensitivities to help them. Thus the paradigm is one that has potential to grow and spontaneously expand on itself. In this manner patients are often proselytized while they are being healed and recover by becoming healers. The process is embedded in an ideological system that provides a rationalization for what has happened, thus generating a healing cult such as that offered by Spiritism in Puerto Rico.

The subject matter and integrative purpose of this book will prove relevant to a broad spectrum of readers. Mental health professionals, psychiatry residents, and medical students will find the manifestations of familiar DSMIIIR[2] mental disorders and their treatment in another culture enlightening. Anthropologists, particularly medical anthropologists, will find here a practical application of their discipline in helping develop more therapeutic approaches to the care of the mentally ill in settings such as Puerto Rico. This book may also offer new insights to scholars of religious studies who have an interest in the spiritual dimensions of healing, as well as to those who might still be convinced of the mystical aspects of healing.

Edward F. Foulks, M.D., Ph.D.
Sellars-Polchow Professor
Department of Psychiatry and Neurology
Tulane University School of Medicine

Notes

1. Mircea Eliade, *Myths, Dreams, and Mysteries: The Encounter Between Contemporary Faiths and Archaic Realities,* trans. P. Mairet (New York: Harper and Row, 1960).
2. American Psychiatric Association, *Diagnostic and Statistical Manual of Mental Disorders,* 3d rev. ed. (Washington, D.C.: APA, 1987).

Preface

On Having Been Called:
A Very Personal Note

When I began this book, a friend said, "Why are you writing this book? There's always a reason." There is a very important reason, of course. My work with the *Espiritistas* completely changed my life. It led to a search for completeness at a time when I was fragmented and changing. My understanding came slowly because their messages were veiled in strange metaphors. As was my way, I denied such deep, emotionally charged meanings. In fact, I had sacrificed a great part of myself to becoming a "social scientist," so that I learned to think habitually in a logical, straightforward way. I was able to marshal arguments that could convince even the most talented of thinkers.

It was many years before I was even dimly aware that I had sacrificed anything. This realization came only after I was groomed, for a third time, to become a Spiritist medium. I was regularly being told by healers that I had been ordained to be a healer and must try to submit to spiritual forces, both within and without. I followed their advice, for the sake of my research, and allowed myself to fall under their tutelage. This was most gratifying because I was able to share the feelings of well-being that attended their clients' relief from distress. However, several times I became frightened, especially once when my consciousness began to alter and I slipped away while attending a healing session. Happily (I thought at the time), a friend grabbed my shoulders and shook me back to ordinary consciousness. On another occasion, I was put at the table on behalf of a healer who was a friend and enjoined to "see" into the water. I had a vision of her laid out in a coffin, surrounded by her family. I refused to reveal the vision, either to her or to others attending that session, and resolved not to try again.

Some years later in Puerto Rico, I underwent formal training in a group led by a famous *Espiritista*. Shortly afterward, a crisis arose in my own life. Instead of letting my intuition and feelings guide me, I tried to be "rational." This resulted in years of suffering but also in the dim awareness that I *had* to recover that part of myself that was arational; I had to trust that part of myself that *felt* things and to permit feelings to guide my movements through life. Whether because of my position as principal investigator of a project sponsored by the Department of Health of Puerto Rico or because I could not permit myself to go into that twilight state in which all mediums work, I was never able to do spirit work. In the end I was forced to submit to my academic persona, which persisted as observer and interpreter. However, I had found an avenue of awareness into myself, which was later to be broadened by psychoanalytic training.

The twin messages of Spiritist healing are available to everyone who can understand: only in pain can one find lost parts of oneself, and one must submit and wait for direction and understanding rather than force or control the direction in which important events proceed and solutions emerge. In writing this book I have submitted to my inner voices and to those of various spirits—probably, but not certainly, one and the same.

Although this is an ethnographic study, based on systematic observations, interviews, and questionnaires—some observations began some twenty-five years ago in the context of a study of Puerto Rican migrants to Philadelphia, culminating in the Therapist-Spiritist Training Project in Puerto Rico from July 1976 to June 1980—I have decided not to write in the standard mode found in most ethnographic reports. Instead I wish my very intense personal experience of women as healers and patients in Puerto Rico to speak through the observations and narratives I recount. For this desire, I acknowledge a debt of gratitude to Paul Stoller (1984), whose discussions of the need for ethnographies to bring human "being" to life have greatly influenced my thinking about how to write about the experience of one's field. My own experience of humanity was profoundly affected by all of the healers, but particularly by the Spiritists. They often insisted that this book was meant to be written by spirits who desired its appearance in the visible world. I have gladly accepted the spirits' offer of inspirational influence in the hope that my readers will also experience "beingness" through and with the healers and their clients and patients, as well as through those inspired coworker/friends who shared their own special beingness while working in the Project.

Acknowledgments

As an author and researcher I owe an enormous debt of appreciation to a multitude of friends and coworkers who participated in, or facilitated, the Therapist-Spiritist Project in Puerto Rico. Of those who worked and believed in the Project, Dr. Hector Rivera Lopez, its director during the second and third years and data analyst during the fourth year, is justifiably featured in this book as my co-observer and cointerpreter. Hector's unstinting belief in the Project went beyond all measure of the deep friendship that emerged out of our experiences and still sustains me at times. Edgardo Rivera Saez, the Project's photographer and field-worker during its second and third years, and Fredeswinda Román, a field-worker during the third year and chief data analyst and hardworking assistant on the films, deserve special mention.

Without them the Project and the dissemination of its results simply would not have reached fulfillment. I still count them among my best-loved friends, to whom I owe a great debt. Of the many persons who both worked and participated in the Project, the help, wisdom, and love of Spiritists Don Jorge Quevedo, Doña Luisa Mora Carmona, Doña Guané Clara de Millán, Doña Dominga Vasquez, Doña Santa Gonzalez, Doña Estefanía Rosario Ruiz, Doña Belgica Negron, Doña Geraldina Pou, Doña Lucía Neris, Doña Carmen Búsigo, Don Tranquilino Cruz, Don Marcial Figueroa, and Doña Palmira Ramos went beyond any expectations. Other Spiritist participants who helped enormously were Don Moncho Román Felix, Don Pedro Millán Clara, and Doña Encarnación Villefañe, now deceased. In the Department of Health of Puerto Rico, the former subsecretary for mental health, Dr. José Nuñez Lopez, was indispensable at the initiation of the Project and provided excellent guidance and support during its first year. Dr. Luis Guillermo de Jesus, then regional director of the Caguas Region, made our second and third years possible and provided excellent advice. Drs. Luis Enrique Morales III, José Gomez Blanco, Carlos Robles, and Lydia Brugueras offered support, advice, and many new perspectives. Therapists who generously gave information and support were Señora Carmen Julia, Señor Benjamín Rosa, Señora Cándida González de Baez, Señor Daniel Berrios, and Señoras Naida Grin, Nitza Colon, Nereida Rosa Morales, Evelyn Santiago, Sonia Flecha, and Aurea Bonilla. Two secretaries of health of the Commonwealth of Puerto Rico, Dr. Jaime Rivera Dueño and Dr. Luis Izquierda Mora, gave their official support and ratified the sponsorship of the Department of Health. Among many excellent lecturers were Drs. Tomás Blanco and Juan Moran. Dr. Michael A. Woodbury was especially helpful and gave support and help beyond what was requested. Two busy scholar-researchers generously acted as invaluable consultants: Dr. Eugene B. Brody, secretary general of the World Federation for Mental Health; and Dr. Robert Goldsmith, professor at the School of Medicine, University of California at San Francisco. The National Institute of Mental Health, Division of Manpower Research and Training, funded the Therapist-Spiritist Training Project in Puerto Rico (MH14310–03 and MH 15210). I remain grateful to them as to all who so generously helped.

To all those mentioned above and to many others, I owe a huge debt of appreciation. And there are still others who helped with the preparation of the data and the manuscript that I must acknowledge. Dr. Richard Harris of the Department of Psychology at the University of New Mexico was extremely patient and generous with his skills as a statistician. He provided the statistical approach that made the comparisons across healing systems possible. Kellie Masterson, my editor at Westview Press, not only made publication possible but transformed the difficult time of finishing the manuscript into one of pleasure and fun. Kellie's talents reach far beyond editing; they belong to a category I label "humanity" because they represent special warmth, love, and encouragement. Dr. Edward F. Foulks spent much time carefully reading and giving a critique of the manuscript, proving himself a true friend as well as an excellent scholar. I am honored that he wrote the Foreword. Helga Umpierre of Puerto Rico also graciously gave of her valuable time in reading and criticizing the manuscript. Finally, I want to thank my husband, Craig C. Chioino. Because of his love and encouragement, he not only successfully carried out seemingly impossible and onerous tasks of data management and analysis but also provided assistance and patience throughout the period leading to and during the writing of this book.

Joan Koss-Chioino

1

The Setting and the Subjects

This is really a schizophrenic society. Puerto Ricans have two languages, two citizenships, two basic philosophies of life, two flags, two anthems, two loyalties. It is very hard for human beings to deal with all this ambivalence.

—Rene Marques, quoted in Wagenheim, *Puerto Rico*

Wisdom and love walk together.

—An *Espiritista* in Puerto Rico, 1977

I have been writing this book for many years, although without putting words on paper. The fervor and commitment of the healers I have known, both medical and traditional, have inspired the task. Their womanliness and special strength while they struggle with adversity are incredibly attractive; observing them at work has touched the deepest layers of my being. However, it is difficult to understand them or their work without describing the sociocultural context in which they live and carry out their healing mission. Following this description, I introduce the Therapist-Spiritist Training Project, which was the context in which we all came together as well as the vehicle for the many encounters and events narrated in this book.

Puerto Rico at the End of the Twentieth Century

Given its geopolitical importance, it may be surprising that Puerto Rico is a small island, approximately one hundred by thirty-five miles at its widest and longest points. It lies almost midway between North and South America—geographically, economically, and in terms of its lifestyle. However, its warm, crowded, extroverted, Spanish-speaking ambience shows its closest relationships to be with other Caribbean countries.

Puerto Rico has lived under the political domination of the United States since 1898, acquired by the United States when Spain ceded both it and the Philippines in the Treaty of Paris as the result of the Spanish-American War. Although there have been sporadic independence movements over two centuries, Puerto Ricans have actually mobilized only one revolution, known as the *Grito de Lares* (Cry of Lares), in 1868. This attempt to be free of Spanish colonial domination was extremely short-lived. In 1898 the island passed almost unobserved from being a Spanish to being a U.S. colony. Its political status changed again in 1952 to that of a commonwealth, a "Free Associated State" (*Estado Libre Asociado*). Since that time it has governed its own internal affairs but is still subject to U.S. laws and policies for external matters. Puerto Rico's Spanish heritage has remained ascendant, tempered—even somewhat eroded—by the addition of African peoples and traditions during the eighteenth and nineteenth centuries and by the increasing impact of North American lifeways and the English language in the twentieth century.

Approximately 3.5 million people inhabit the island. Another 1.5 million, who identify themselves as Puerto Ricans and Neoricans, can be found in the continental United States. Of these, most are in the Northeast, but many reside in other regions, mostly east of the Mississippi River. Because Puerto Rico is part of the United States and no international boundaries obstruct passage between the island and the mainland, Puerto Ricans and "continentals" travel easily back and forth and may also settle in one place or the other for brief periods or many years. Currently, two generations of Puerto Rican children have grown up in New York City and nearby northeastern towns and cities. These people, poised between two cultures and speaking two languages, are known as Neoricans, or Niuyorricans. As adults some decide to live in Puerto Rico and thus have hastened the inevitable flow of culture change on the island itself. However, they have retained the main outlines of their Latin attitudinal and belief systems, folk religious practices, and patterns of familial relationships as well as identity as Puerto Ricans (Rodriguez-Cortes, 1990). Although they speak Spanish as well as English, many are unable to read or write their parents' and grandparents' native language. Some patterns of social behavior have changed—in particular, gender relationships and sex roles.

The most important sources of social and cultural change in Puerto Rico have been the development of an industrialized economy and the related wholesale acceptance of the high value of middle-class status, patterned on the North American model. This has strongly affected men's and women's roles as a result of the new attitude that a woman's place is no longer confined to the home. Middle-class status is contingent upon higher education for both sexes and the expectation that women will contribute their wages to domestic incomes. However, this far-reaching change in gender roles and expectations is only one outcome of a complex history of U.S. economic and political policies toward its colony. Another important result is that Puerto Rico possesses a nebulous political status that can only be resolved by an act of Congress following a plebiscite that specifies the will of the people for statehood or independence or a continuation of commonwealth status. Up to the present the people's will has been to continue their commonwealth relationship; however, a plebiscite has been discussed by the local government and the U.S. Congress. Popular sentiment is reported to favor statehood, but Congress has been indecisive.

Intimately related to the lack of resolution of its political status is the fact that Puerto Rico is highly dependent upon the United States for its present standard of living, the highest among Latin American countries. However, the economic benefit of U.S. development of the island's economy in the mid-twentieth century, away from monoagricultural exports and toward factory-produced goods with a guaranteed market, has been much diluted in the 1980s. This is due to the legislated decline in tax incentives for U.S. investors, who are consequently searching for cheaper labor in less-developed Caribbean countries. Puerto Rico's high standard of living has in part been rescued by federal transfers (social welfare and other benefits) but has also been periodically cramped by free-enterprise policies governing trade with the United States and by fluctuations of the U.S. economy. Immigration to the continental United States has continued to reduce the island's overcrowded, job-seeking population but has recently become merely a raising of the lid of poverty to let off the pressure-building steam of economic distress. In addition, migration opens the door for the transfer of many negative aspects of northeastern U.S. urban life, such as drug trafficking, substance abuse, and sexually transmitted diseases.

From Economic to Social Change: A Tale of Two Cultures

As numerous writers point out, describing Puerto Rican "culture" is a difficult task, given both its contradictions and its dual tendencies: Puerto Rico has one face looking backward toward a not-so-glorious, Spanish colonial past heavy with poverty, and another anxiously peering into an uncertain, Americanized future, poor in tradition but richer in consumer goods (see Lewis, 1963; Wagenheim, 1970; Nieves Falcon, 1973; Carr, 1985; Pico, 1986). Some authors, such as Pico (1986), seem to view the Americanization of the island as a logical consequence of economic growth, but others, such as Carr (1985), talk about the "clash" of the two cultures. Carr points out that writers and political leftists idealize the old traditions, while denying the poverty and oppression formerly suffered by *campesinos* (peasants). Yet it has been amply demonstrated that most Puerto Ricans are willing to trade their colonial past for a more comfortable present, even if it includes neocolonial status. Rather than conflict being a leitmotiv of Puerto Rican social life, ambivalence and contradiction seem to be the major themes, resulting in abundant confusion as to the direction and meaning of life. This situation has been aptly labeled "unstable hybridization," an uncomfortable cultural dualism (Carr, 1985).

Social and cultural changes have been far-reaching in some directions. For example, the traditional two-class structure of rich and poor has disappeared, and most Puerto Ricans identify with the democratic ideal of a monoclass society where everyone benefits from free enterprise and widely accessible consumerism. (Vocal but few, members of the socialist political parties are exceptions in terms of their views, but not always in terms of their behavior.) A dual set of public holidays is celebrated; U.S. patriots and Puerto Rican historical figures share the yearly calendar. Celebrations of the Spanish feast of the Three Kings on January 6 follow closely upon a lavish, media-driven Christmas, sans snow. In other areas of life "hybridization" is not as even-handed in its effects. Although the general structure of family relationships and associated values, such as an organic interdependence of persons within nuclear and extended families resulting in lifetime (and beyond) closeness of blood ties, has been preserved, emigration has affected family life in many negative ways. Among its direct and indirect effects are continuing increases in alcoholism, drug use and associated crime, family violence, divorce and mother-headed families, physical and sexual abuse of children, and sexually transmitted diseases. The prevalence of AIDS, for example, is one of the highest reported among countries in the Western hemisphere (50.7 per 100,000 in 1990). This high rate is due in part to gay sons returning home when almost moribund with the disease. Deaths from heart disease (the leading cause) and homicide also show a steady increase through the 1980s. These indicators of social distress and chaos can only be attributed in part to migration. They are also attributable to the societal disorganization and anomie that seem to increase with each passing year, somewhat balanced by social development in terms of expansion of institutions for higher learning and educational opportunities, more activities in the arts, and widespread involvement in political issues.

Puerto Rican Paradoxes: Gender and Relationship

In my descriptions of medical and traditional healers in Puerto Rico and their patients and clients, I address the thorny issue of women in trouble in a society that scarcely recognizes the deep difficulties its way of life creates. Having lived that life for years, I am certain that no particular set of institutions or mores can be blamed. However, there are many difficult contradictions in Puerto Rican social life, such as a poorly integrated bundle of outmoded and newer traditions about male and female roles and relationships, a spurious economic system that requires everyone to be a wage earner but offers limited opportunities to women, and increasing instability in family and community organization at a time when women are most in need of supportive networks.

Unfortunately this "woman's tragedy" is not unique to Puerto Rico. The social and economic conditions that have nourished it in Puerto Rico have generated similar effects in the continental United States for at least two decades, particularly among poor women. In Latin America and the Caribbean, as countries enter a period of rapid economic development and cultural change, the traditional subordination of women by men leads to inequality and sexism in the workplace. Yet women's issues are submerged by problems in labor relations, family disruption, and unequal distribution of income, as well as by extensive crime and substance abuse. Therefore, women's problems are even more difficult to solve because of their underground quality. This situation parallels the relative invisibility of women in the power structure. In the tightly structured, yet rapidly changing, society of Puerto Rico, greatly influenced by North American values and institutions, we find a caricature of the intense social drama of women's lives found in the United States.

Marital relations are at the heart of the changes in gender relations. Traditionally it has been said that men are of the streets (*de las calles*) and women belong at home (*de la casa*). Men have generally sought to control their wives' behavior, particularly with regard to activities outside the home. This pervasive attitude has had to undergo some change, given the dependence upon women's wages and the acceptance of women as wage earners. In direct contrast, men have always been considered "free" to do almost anything they wish, which can include philandering, having a mistress (referred to as a "woman on the left"), and partying away from home (sometimes for days) without notice to their wives and families.

A number of studies on marital relations in Puerto Rico describe how women actually expect such behavior from men. Lopez Garriga (1980) lists the adjectives her lower- and middle-class female subjects used to describe men. Of the sixteen used most frequently, only four were positive. The first and second choices of one-third of the respondents were "*dominante*" and "*machista*" (chauvinistic), followed by positive adjectives like "good fathers and husbands," "good providers," and "responsible." "Irresponsible," "immature," "egotist," and "not very understanding" were other adjectives that were popular in describing the very negative feelings of women toward their men. Women often view men as immature and demanding by nature and assert that they must be treated with care and manipulated—much as one tries to control a wayward child who is too big and powerful to spank (Safa, 1974). Yet Puerto Rican society "perceives women as emotional and dependent, whose lives revolve around the desires and actions of their men" (Lopez Garriga, 1980:185).

The actuality of male power and authority in Puerto Rican society is an established fact, as is the stated need of Puerto Rican women to acquire more powerful positions for decisionmaking in their own lives. This need creates a contradiction for those women who have achieved professional positions, earn good salaries, and contribute significantly to the finances of their upwardly mobile, middle-class families. As Lopez Garriga's (1980) study shows, these women try to resolve the contradictions in their roles by employing more diverse and manipulative strategies than do lower-class women, whose opportunities for work and financial independence are less extensive and rewarding.

However, middle-class, professional women (and also many lower-class, employed women) are less likely to prolong their suffering in marriage (two out of five marriages end in divorce). Even other women seem more adept than women used to be at employing strategies to manipulate their husbands in the service of satisfying some of their own needs. One study demonstrates that more married than divorced women feel they have help from husbands with household chores and more decision-making power in their marriages (Muñoz Vásquez, 1980). The study describes divorced women as having suffered significantly more abuse, often because of the effects of alcoholism on the behavior of their former husbands. Despite these partial remedies to an endemic situation of female subordination and unhappiness in marriage, a high toll is exacted in terms of emotional distress and associated mental and physical illness in women.

Marcia Rivera Quintero (1980) sees the effect of this drama as change, even in the ways women perceive themselves. The situation created by sociocultural changes provides a context for the surfacing of important facets of personhood and social behavior. The descriptions in this book, of women struggling with illness either as healers or as patients, are a record of the drama of women's lives, more exciting than the TV novellas (soap operas) to which so many are addicted. This book aims at portraying the experience and context of Puerto Rican womanhood in all of its complex, heroic, yet quite imperfect, reality. Illness events provide us with a mirror on women (to paraphrase the famous anthropologist Clyde Kluckholn) in their basic roles as nurturers and counselors in Puerto Rican society. When illness events are interpreted by either sufferer or healer, they generally offer views of the dark side of the experience of femininity but also of lighter perspectives on daily life that women hold. Most important, illness events help us understand how women interpret both positive and negative experiences as self-related phenomena. Precisely at times of illness are women most threatened by assaults on their self-esteem and sometimes by the decimation of their very selves.

In all of the Latin American and Caribbean countries for which we have data, women as healers receive other women's (and men's) distress. Whether formally trained in the helping professions or a recipient of a sacred trust passed on to them by a beloved grandmother, aunt, or godmother and called a "gift from God," their healing practice is a special outcome of a particularly feminine element of being. Whether as much-sought-after grandmothers, wise in the ways of folk remedies as well as in the ways of the world, or as cult adherents, tightly bound to groups that undergo ecstatic trance and are possessed by African gods or Catholic saints, women find that healing is the connective tissue between them and their knowing themselves. This knowing is mediated by a feminine compulsion both to receive and to affiliate.

D. W. Winnicott (1971) identified three aspects of the feminine element of being (as cited in Ulanov, 1981:77): "being as being-at-the-core-of-oneself; being as beginning of being-with-one-another; and being as possessed of a personal continuity." Just as the infant gradually comes to know herself as a separate oneness with her mother, who mirrors her being, healer and patient come to know themselves as women through "being-with-each-other." I am especially indebted to Ann Ulanov (1981) for her concept of the "receiving woman" and her discussion of how one can experience "being-at-one-with" during therapy as a necessary prologue to knowing one's self. I would extend her idea that the therapist reflects the self the patient brings to her session to the idea that the patient also reflects the therapist's self, although this is not always acknowledged by either one. When both are women, within whom the feminine is constantly active, they are given an experience of their feminine selves.

Background of the Therapist-Spiritist Project

The main goal of the Therapist-Spiritist Project was to design and carry out programs that would create a bridge between conventional biomedical health care—mental health care in particular—and the popular healing system, *Espiritismo.* One might ask, "Why sponsor or fund such an effort?" To answer, it is necessary to give a few facts about the recent history of the mental health movement and the role of social science in that movement. By the early 1970s social scientists had become aware of the applied potentialities of widespread medical pluralism, including traditional healing both in developing nations and in first-world countries like the United States. Anthropologists have always studied nonmedical, indigenous healing systems. However, prior to the mid-1960s, ethnomedical practices were labeled "religious" phenomena and described from that perspective. Few anthropologists highlighted the medical aspects of healing beliefs and practices or appreciated them as valid alternatives or complements to Western biomedical health care. Yet healing beliefs and practices were recognized as important, culturally patterned psychological phenomena (Wallace, 1966). In my earlier studies of Puerto Rican *Espiritismo* during the 1960s, I explored its sociopsychological and historical dimensions rather than its societal role as a community-based, indigenous mental health and health care system (Koss, 1965, 1972, 1976).

The institutionalization of community-based mental health care delivery began in the early 1960s with the U.S. Community Mental Health Centers Act of 1963. The Act carried with it the ideal that everyone is entitled to mental health services regardless of where they live or whether they can pay for the services. Although the federal government defined the essential and desirable activities of a community mental health center, the Act also described how the states (and Puerto Rico) would insure that community mental health centers would provide comprehensive services. The central idea was to base mental health clinics in local communities, which in turn would find suitable property, raise money needed beyond the government's allotment, locate sources of ongoing funding to run the center, plan the details of the building, and develop the center's program components. In addition, it was mandated that a community board would oversee the program with regard to its meeting federal standards. The mental health center was to be established in a locale that would meet the requirement of a geographically defined "catchment area" of between 75,000 and 200,000 people. The mobilization of outreach programs involving institutional liaisons with schools, welfare agencies, the justice system, and nongovernmental institutions such as churches and nursing homes had to be included. The Act mandated twenty-four-hour emergency services for persons with acute episodes of mental disorder and day hospitalization for those with long-term psychiatric illness. In addition to ambulatory services, the community mental health center was required to have a research and development component, focused on both prevention and continual assessment of community needs and problems.

Once the community approach to mental health care delivery was institutionalized, assessments of the role of informal institutions in the mental health of a community revealed that popular healing systems were frequently used for mental health crises and continuity of care. It was confirmed that persons in emotional crises frequently used the services of folk healers, either simultaneously with biomedical health care or as a first resort. During the 1970s the National Institute of Mental Health encouraged and funded a number of projects aimed not only at research into traditional healing in ethnic minority communities but also at exploring the use of healing services offered by traditional healers.[1] A few projects had the practical goal of interchange and bridging the gap between the formal biomedical health care system and the traditional, informal alternative.[2] Foremost among them was the School for Medicine Men project in which young Navahos were trained to become medicine men, and they and older medicine men were enrolled in programs in which medical doctors provided scientific data on diagnosis and treatment in Western biomedicine.

The widespread use of Spiritism in Puerto Rico and by Puerto Ricans in the United States had been recognized in the 1960s by Rogler and Hollingshead (1961, 1965), by Koss (1965), and by Garrison (1977a). These early studies focused largely on descriptions of how healers worked. In later publications Garrison (1977a, 1977b) systematically examined clients' complaints. She, Harwood (1977), and Koss (1975) compared similarities and differences between how psychiatrists and Spiritists work at healing, but did not present systematic material on clients' experience of suffering or specific information on how Spiritist clients utilized and responded to mental health care services.

The Puerto Rican Department of Health, Division of Mental Health, was well aware of the role of Spiritism in communities in its catchment areas. In 1971, after I had carried out several studies of Spiritism in Puerto Rico, I was hired as a consultant and in-service trainer for mental health workers in the community mental health centers. Not only did the subsecretary for mental health at that time endorse the community mental health model but, like other medical doctors and health professionals, he had relatives who believed in Spiritism. He once told us how his wife's emotionally disturbed uncle, a Vietnam veteran, had been "cured" by an *Espiritista* after several psychiatrists had failed to help him. One outcome of my work with the Health Department of Puerto Rico was an invitation by a project officer of the National Institute of Mental Health to write a proposal for a project aimed at developing a formal bridge between the community mental health system and Spiritism.

The general objectives of the initial proposal for the Therapist-Spiritist Training Project were (1) to establish a forum for the meaningful exchange of information between the two healing systems (this was later expanded to include primary care physicians, particularly those in training), (2) to offer a training curriculum to provide knowledge and skills to the members of each system, and (3) to develop new psychotherapeutic approaches from a synthesis of the most relevant and effective healing techniques in each system.

Once the project was funded, groups of Spiritist healers and health professionals met in seminars for six hours per week during three ten-month academic years in three catchment areas of the western (largest) health region in Puerto Rico. For two years the seminars were based in the Community Mental Health Centers (CMHC), with a few participants from nearby hospitals and public health clinics (*Centros de Diagnostico y Tratamiento*, or CDT). The third year's program was based in a regional public health hospital and coordinated with the CMHC of the community. Well-known Spiritist healers and health professionals from the staffs of seven public health institutions were recruited during the spring and summer prior to each seminar program. Three additional programs of six months' duration in each area were attended by medical residents and some of their attending physicians, as well as by Spiritists and mental health paraprofessionals.

Information on the Project's participants was collected and included sociodemographic data, health status, life history, measures assessing the participant's views and treatment of clients/patients, and beliefs and attitudes toward the two types of healing systems. In addition, information on the clients/patients of each participant over one-month periods, prior to and following participation in the Project's seminar program, was compiled, and pre- and post-treatment interviews of two new clients/patients of each participant were carried out and recorded. Many health professionals, community leaders, and Spiritists attended the seminars as guests, but complete dossiers of information were compiled on seventeen women mental health professionals and seven young women medical doctors, eleven male mental health professionals and twenty male medical doctors. Although these participants are collectively referred to in this book as "therapists," where differences are relevant I discuss them separately. Dossiers of information were also compiled on Spiritist core participants—thirty-five women and thirteen men.

The seminars consisted of two types of "courses" held each week. The first was a conference that included two lecturers—a health professional and a Spiritist healer. The second weekly session centered on discussion of a case seen in the CMHC or public health clinics, compared with a matched case seen by a Spiritist healer. The scheduled content of the weekly conferences varied according to the interests of the medical, psychological, or Spiritist lecturers we recruited for a particular lecture series.[3] The schedule for the lecture/discussions from January to May 1979, for example, began with a lecture by me on anthropological perspectives on health and illness and a discussion of concepts of "community health." This was matched by a lecture by Doña Guane, one of our first participants, on health and illness from the Spiritist viewpoint. The lecture/discussion session the following week, and for the next three weeks, included two lecturers—a health professional and a Spiritist—who discussed therapeutic techniques in each healing system. The sixth week's meeting was the beginning of a four-week series on psychopharmacology and herbal medicine as applied to diseases/illnesses of the central nervous system, the cardiovascular system, and the digestive system. Following this series, a two-week series in April examined the referral system in the biomedical treatment of emotional disorders and other illnesses as compared to referrals made by Spiritists across their diagnostic categories. During the first week in May all of the participants met at a Spiritist *centro* (healing center) headed by one of them. The remaining three weeks of that program were dedicated to lectures on organic brain syndromes and equivalent conceptualizations and diagnoses by the Spiritists, as well as to lectures on psychosomatic illness and views on developmental life stages and illness from both medical and Spiritist perspectives.

For the sessions in which cases were reviewed each week we asked various participants to prepare cases for presentation and then chose a presenter from the opposite healing system to match the case with one of her own. Sometimes the presenting complaints were matched; at other times it was the gender and age of the patients or clients that were matched. We did not dictate the type of case or guide the process of matching because we wished to allow the specific perspectives of each system to emerge. We did assist the Spiritists in developing a general format for preparing their case presentations but left it vague enough to allow them to express their special views and idioms. In fact, these presentations seemed to take on a life of their own, even though they roughly conformed to the usual case presentation format.

One conference series was held in the regional hospital of Humacao, the base headquarters of the Project in 1979. Almost all of the seminar meetings were held in public health settings, either hospitals or mental health centers. It was originally planned to rotate each week to a Spiritist *centro*. However, this proved impractical, and we held only occasional meetings there. The disadvantage to the Spiritists in terms of comfort and recognition seemed outweighed by the prestige and legitimization that meeting in medical institutions lent to the Project's activities. Because Spiritist practices had been denigrated for decades by authorities in the biomedical system, as well as by the Catholic Church, the Spiritists' initial lack of ease in a public health setting was offset by the setting's symbolic value in highlighting the fact that their presence and participation in the Project had official sanction in the medical community.

The Project not only permitted the collection of invaluable facts that allowed a direct comparison of biomedical and traditional perspectives on a variety of topics and case approaches but was also the beginning of a long, fruitful dialogue (that I hope will assist the emergence of better ways to deal with health and mental health problems in Puerto Rico). It also provided an important opportunity for healers to know each other and share life experiences. For most of the participants, these experiences were different depending on whether they were health professionals, physicians, or Spiritist healers. This book will describe both the important differences and the similarities. In the discussion to follow, I introduce the healers in the context of their very different institutions and systems of medical and traditional healing practices.

The reader may wonder at the use of the word *healer* to include mental health workers, nurses, social workers, and physicians with folk healers. Most Spiritist participants had very little formal education but worked intensively at traditional healing and its study as an avocation. The mental health professionals who took part in the seminar programs had four- or six-year university educations and were beginning new, modern careers in mental health care delivery. Most of the young female physicians who participated in our project were beginning the last year of a long educational journey into medicine and were about to take on the high-status professional role they had justly earned. Although the contrasts between these two groups of women are great, the experience of being a woman and a healer often transcended the differences in surprising ways. After becoming acquainted through the Therapist-Spiritist Project, many of the health professionals entered into friendships with Spiritist healers and informally consulted them about their own and patients' problems. It was as if the recognition of an important common concern acted as a strong, natural bond between women and men possessed of an intense interest in receiving and helping others, regardless of how and where they had received their training.

Spiritism: A Popular Healing System

The tripartite ethos of sociality, hospitality, and receptivity to expressed feelings, both one's own and those of others, is central to Puerto Rican culture. Puerto Rican life is mainly made up of people and intimate relationships. Yet Puerto Rico has always been a crossroads for streams of immigrant peoples, as well as a site of rapid change in lifeways and political programs. The societal uncertainty about materialistic and scientific philosophies and the difficult colonial relations of the latter part of the nineteenth century provided a context for the ready acceptance of a new "scientific" and "philosophic" religion from France—Spiritism. It was introduced into Puerto Rico by intellectuals studying in Paris and Madrid. Believers avow that Spiritism was "given" to the world sometime prior to 1853 through spirits communicating with Leon Hippolyte Denizarth Rivail (1803–1869), a French scholar and magnetist working with other distinguished French academics. Rivail's interest in spirit phenomena had been aroused by the popular response in England to the Fox sisters' discovery of spirit rappings in upper New York State, a wave of interest and exploration of the spirit realm that became known in the English-speaking world as Spiritualism.

Rivail published seven books under the pen name Allan Kardec. The first of these was *The Spirits' Book* (1886), first published in Paris, perhaps as early as 1853. Although the book was distinctly Christian in its ideological focus, Rivail proposed a new "science" that began with an exploration of a newly discovered dimension of spiritual existence (Kardec, 1883). He believed every individual to have a personal spirit that passes over to the spirit world at the death of the material body; this spirit then exists in a parallel spirit world awaiting reincarnation. The spirit's corporeal life is an opportunity for spiritual evolution through good deeds and moral behavior. Those who suffer (*una prueba*, "test") during their incarnations are paying for the misdeeds of an earlier life. However, one's current life can be used as an opportunity to evolve. Evolution of the spirit can be assisted by one's guardian angel or special protectors (*guías protectores*), who are called upon through prayer to assist the living in their trials and tribulations. Everyone has the potential for "developing their faculties" to communicate with the spirit world; those who "develop" become mediums by uncovering the identities of their spirit protectors and learning how to assist other persons to communicate with spirits. Mediums and believers who regularly attend *centros* are called *Espiritistas.*

The apparently rapid spread of Spiritism in Puerto Rico during the latter part of the nineteenth century was in part due to the disenfranchisement of popular folk healers, who dispensed herbs and prayers, acted as midwives, and called upon the saints to mediate with the ever-distant and often punitive Lord of the Universe to aid those suffering physical or emotional ills (Koss, 1976). Spiritism was a new wave of ideas, very similar to those that preceded, but now legitimized and codified by a set of texts on how to intercede in the spirit world and supported by beliefs phrased in new "scientific" language. *Curanderos* (curers), *sobadores* (massage-curers), and *comadronas* (midwives) were being attacked by the Catholic Church and also by the *protomedicates,* the licensing boards established in 1844 by the Spanish colonial government. The Spiritist medium took over the social role of the *curandero* (or rather the latter became an *Espiritista*). Spiritists preserved most of the *curanderos*' notions about healing by acting as intermediaries with spirits (instead of saints), both those who are bad, or "undeveloped," and bring harm to the living and those who are enlightened and wish to come through to aid loved ones from this or a former existence.

Espiritistas diagnose the causes of illness and other problems but do not directly "heal." Healing can occur when the spirit medium assists the sufferer to come into harmony with the spirit world so as to change his or her physical condition, emotions, way of life, or destiny. Those spirit mediums who are very successful counsel patients on how to relate to significant others and instruct them on the "real" meaning of life. Spirit mediums are self-selected and have had very special, ecstatic experiences of spirits early in their lives. They carry out their work as an avocation and usually do not ask for payment, because to do so would mean the loss of their mediumistic faculties and capacity to help others. They practice their profession in the evenings or on weekends, if employed, and can be especially active during retirement years when their labors as mothers, teachers, nurses, office or factory workers have ceased. Many have been seriously ill, both emotionally and physically, but have overcome their illnesses and learned the most important of life's lessons—when to challenge adversity and when to accept disability as inevitable. All of the *Espiritistas* I know work very hard at study and prayer in order to be healers, although they lack licenses and prerogatives. Their course of "development" can be described as a self-selected but indirect relationship with the Holy Spirit, who governs everyone's destiny (Koss, 1975). One's own spirit (*el propio ser*) develops over many lifetimes from a base, ignorant state; instincts change to wisdom and "pure" sentiments, such as love for all beings in the world and enlightenment through spiritual knowledge.

The special life course of these folk healers has much in common with that of their counterparts in other areas of the world. We might call them "urban *curanderos*," as did Press in the *Journal of Health and Social Behavior* (1969) when he described healers in Bogota, Colombia. Popular healers are found in all Puerto Rican communities, and most of them practice some brand of spirit mediumship. Currently, *Santería*, a religious healing cult imported from Cuba, has a growing number of devotees among both Cubans exiled to the island and Puerto Ricans.

Few of the many studies of shamanic healers convey the sense of dedication, love, and fortitude that emanates from most of these healers at work. This is not to imply that they always successfully heal (that is, meet their own or clients' expectations for relief) or that none are charlatans professing to be "true" *Espiritistas* without following the strict ethical and moral understandings of the majority who "work" at Spiritism.

Shamanic healers in other parts of the world are initiated into their healing avocations through life crises such as serious illness (Lewis, 1971). They may learn their healing techniques through apprenticeship to other healers but are usually "called" to develop themselves as healers by special, non-human beings (or "spirits") who appear during illness crises. *Espiritistas* in Puerto Rico frequently experience their calling during childhood when they receive communications from nonliving beings. The capacities to receive images of the invisible spirit world and to willingly enter into and control altered states of consciousness are two important aspects of becoming a medium and dedicating one's life to helping others.

Community-based Mental Health Care

Because Puerto Rico participates in all of the major health programs developed by the United States, it receives the mandates and benefits of the Community Mental Health Act of 1963. During the 1960s and 1970s, eleven community mental health centers were established. The Therapist-Spiritist Project focused its programs on three centers: Caguas, Cayey, and Humacao. Although over fifty women on the staffs of the mental health centers and other health care agencies attended our seminars, detailed information was collected on only twenty-two women who worked at the mental health centers or at coordinating agencies and who participated regularly in the Project's programs. These women included three who were nurses at mental health centers and five who worked at district hospitals, three social workers, seven "psychosocial technicians" (mental health workers), two psychologists, and two health care administrators.

These mental health professionals were relatively young, ranging in age from early twenties to early forties, part of a new wave of health professionals working in the mental health field within a public health setting. Very few had been trained specifically for their positions, but all were imbued with a desire to alleviate the patients' problems. All but two of the mental health workers described here were counselors or psychotherapists or workers in day care or hospitalization units. In contrast to the Spiritist healers, their work took place during specific hours; they were free for family life after 5:00 PM each day. Even so, many of these women saw their patients after working hours and sought special training experiences after work (such as the seminars of the Therapist-Spiritist Project). For the most part, their motivation to deal with the human tragedy they encountered daily was quite high. They also encountered difficulties in their vocations, but in ways quite different from the *Espiritistas*. Job-related suffering came largely from frustration over lack of knowledge of how to reverse the symptoms of severely emotionally disturbed clients. They tried very hard to deal with complex problems that patients presented but often felt inadequate to intervene in ways that would have lasting effects.

Physicians

Seven women physicians at a district hospital participated in the Project and contributed information on their early lives and current work. These young women appeared quite interested in the idea that they were becoming "healers" as well as physicians. All of the professional women, but especially these young doctors, spoke of the frustration of being unable to change circumstances and settings that caused or contributed to illnesses they were called upon to treat. As a result, they were often receptive to much of what the *Espiritistas* said but carefully evaluated this information against the background of their medical studies. In contrast to many of their male counterparts, these women had family backgrounds in which religion was important; they nurtured ideals regarding human nature and a moral, ethical life.

All of the women doctors spoke of harboring since childhood a desire to help others, but they also had chosen their medical careers with a view of themselves as prestigious professionals, respected by those they sought to help. For them the strong desire for a demanding career seemed to have an inhibiting effect on the ability to control the types of personal problems that all women in Puerto Rico must confront. In this way these young doctors shared a common destiny with other women "healers," a destiny full of pitfalls and problems related to being daughters, wives, and mothers, despite well-defined and successful career paths.

Perhaps this was the source of the attraction healers seemed to feel for each other once they became acquainted, secondary to a deep, mutual appreciation of the others' approach to helping people in pain. It was the recognition of problems held in common as women that helped overcome the barriers of formal education and professional status that separated folk healers from the mental health professionals, and both groups from the physicians.

Summary

The foregoing brief descriptions of social life, politics, and the economy in Puerto Rico are included as an introduction to the sociocultural context within which women as healers work and women as patients suffer. In the chapters that follow, I add more details to situate Puerto Rican women as healers and patients in time and social space.

Chapters 2 through 5 describe and highlight some of the main events and activities of the Therapist-Spiritist Project. These events are recalled largely from the viewpoint of the healers, who are the most prominent narrators. However, I also interject my own interpretations and observations, together with those of Hector Rivera Lopez, the Project's Director. He and I intensively discussed all of the events of the Project in much detail during the three years of the Project's life—and for some years afterward. I present these interpretations as if they occurred simultaneously with the events to which they refer. In Chapter 6 I present my own descriptions and interpretations, together with those from secondary sources, on psychiatric illness in Puerto Rico. In that chapter I describe how the meanings of naturally occurring complaints of women being treated for emotional distress are patterned and associated with particular life events and circumstances unique to, in part, Puerto Rican culture. In Chapters 7 through 10 the perspective changes to that of recalling those events in which patients and clients of the healers were involved, either directly or as the subjects of the case reviews.

Four strands of interpretation and description of experience are intertwined in this book: The first is that of the healers talking about themselves and their work; the second is that of the healers' experience of their patients and clients; the third is that of patients and clients talking about their experiences of distress and illness, as well as associated life events; and the fourth is composed of Hector's and my interpretations, augmented by ideas and notions taken from the literature, regarding events or their contexts that make up the first three strands.

Notes

1. See Garrison, 1977a, and Harwood, 1977, for examples of studies of Spiritism among Puerto Ricans in New York City. With regard to the observations in the text, as well as the life history materials and other observations and conclusions in this book, these healers may not be representative of all women in the formal or informal helping professions in Puerto Rico. They are a self-selected group attracted to our project and its goal of interfacing Spiritism with public health care in Puerto Rico.

Moreover, the sixty-one women whose lives and work are described in this book were selected from those who actively participated in the Project and were also willing to respond to a battery of questionnaires. Their identities are shielded by pseudonyms and by rearrangements of their life events. Information on other Project participants, and on persons interviewed or encountered prior to the Project, parallels the data reported here. It indicates a high degree of comparability as well as similarity between the women in this book and other women in Puerto Rico of approximately the same age and educational background.

2. See Brody, 1973; Ruiz and Langrod, 1976; and Garrison, 1979, for a few examples in the literature.

3. See also Koss, 1980.

2

Backgrounds of the Healers in the Therapist-Spiritist Training Project

Working with personal narratives raises questions about authorship: Whose story is to be told? Whose voice is to be heard?

—Personal Narratives Group, *Interpreting Women's Lives*

Who Becomes a Healer and Why?

One day as we awaited the participants of one of the Project's seminars, Hector and I sought to characterize all of the healers we had recruited for the Project. We shared the idea that the healer role in Puerto Rico is an amplification of the ideal mother role (whether one is male or female, Spiritist, therapist or physician), although this seems less clear for the physicians. However, we acknowledged that this notion was somewhat overgeneralized and immediately observed that there are some important differences between mothers and healers. One difference is that healers have a painful awareness of the negative side of their own personalities. Another is healers' knowledge that their role is a vehicle for containing the negativism and malaise of their patients or clients. Both male and female healers nurture their clients and patients, but their relations with them differ significantly from the idealized "good" mothering that women eternally strive to give their children, especially in terms of healers' lack of indulgence of clients and patients and encouragement of autonomy.

Women who become healers in Puerto Rico outwardly seem much like other women of their age and social groups, yet there are some important ways in which they differ. First, their reports of their early lives most often include a deep concern for the problems and illnesses of other family members. Second, pervasive religious attitudes had been established early in their lives. Third, their life goals had already been defined during childhood. Fourth, they are perhaps more ambitious than other women. Finally, these particular women are especially aware of illnesses they themselves experienced as children.

Facts About Healers: Age, Education, and Families

As we looked around the seminar room, we noticed first the women who worked in the mental health centers and public welfare agencies. Most of them were between twenty-one and forty-one years old. An exception was one social worker who was fifty-six years old and had retired three years earlier but volunteered her services at one of the mental health centers. We noted that the women medical doctors were also young, ranging in age from twenty-seven to thirty-five years and having finished their training within the past five years. In contrast, the Spiritist healers were significantly older than other project participants; they ranged in age from forty to seventy-two years.

All of the mental health workers had had some higher education, varying from three years in a school of nursing to completion of a master's degree in psychology, social work, or health education. And all of the medical doctors had completed or were in a fifth year of medical education (the internship year). They and the mental health workers came from the relatively small group of women in Puerto Rico who have had the benefit of higher education. Yet only a few of their parents had achieved professional status or had university educations.

In thinking about the Spiritists, Hector and I noted that only eleven out of thirty-five had received professional or university educations, although two had received occupational training, one as a practical nurse and the other as a beautician. The older Spiritists had had much less opportunity to acquire professional training because higher education for lower-class people, and especially for women, has only become available in the past twenty-five years. Given their stated desire to achieve some recognition (expressed by all of the *Espiritistas*), it is likely that most of the Spiritists, if they had been born later, would have taken advantage of opportunities for higher education.

Looking around the room, we could see that all of these women, young and old, professional and nonprofessional, shared the special personal characteristics of being extremely energetic and intensely interested in people. Even those Spiritist healers with little formal education used their healing avocations to exercise their intellects and their curiosity about other people's psychologies.

What kind of family life did these women have? In all three groups some were married, some were divorced, and some were single. Of the mental health workers, eight were married and had one to four children, six were divorced with children and had not remarried, and eight were single but planned to marry. (The only confirmed single woman was the retired social worker.) Four of the medical doctors were married (one for the second time) and had one or two children, two doctors had divorced, and one had never married.

Without a doubt, marriage and children were considered by these women to be as important as their career plans, not as obstacles or alternative life patterns. We noted that this agrees with the observations of various authors on Puerto Rican women, such as Acosta-Belen and Sjostrom (1980), who note that although educational opportunities have been equally available to men and women since the 1950s and women have availed themselves of more than their share, women are still relegated to "traditional" female professions. This reinforces a rather rigid distinction between male and female social roles in community and family. It is abundantly clear that few women define themselves in terms of their professional achievements or derive the greater part of their feelings of self-worth from a particular profession or occupation (Hidalgo and Christensen, 1979). In fact, only a small group of relatively young women of my acquaintance in Puerto Rico seem to be able to derive deep personal meaning from their work, yet even they continue to avidly pursue roles as wives and mothers. But again and again Hector and I commented to each other that women healers of all types seemed to take great pride in their healing roles. Healing practices were a very significant source of self-esteem, and for the five participants who had never married, even replaced the self-esteem usually acquired in the roles of wife and mother.

Most of the Spiritist healers were or had been married: twenty were living with their husbands at the time of the Project, five were widowed after long marriages, and five were divorced after marriages of two to fifteen years. Only five Spiritist healers had followed different paths: two had participated in consensual marriages that lasted only a short time; one had chosen a professional career in the early 1950s, suffered a severe scoliosis (curvature of the spine) and had never married; and two women lived together in sisterly intimacy that was rumored to be a lesbian relationship. All of the Spiritists, except the last three and an elderly teacher who had only a brief consensual marriage, had completed rearing their natural or adopted children. Most had one to four children who were now independent, but two older Spiritists had fourteen and eighteen children each.

Hector and I agreed that becoming a traditional healer is not a substitute for maternal fulfillment for most Spiritists. Yet for many it is a way to continue to use their mothering skills in a postmaternal period of life. It is not a substitute for the usual maternal pattern of later life that includes great delight in grandmothering and often full-time care of grandchildren. However, for an older woman, working as a healer is clearly a significant way to work with people instead of retiring to a homebound existence and a shrinking community social life. This was as true for those of the eleven professional women Spiritists who had already retired from teaching or counseling as it was for healers without formal education and careers. For all of the Spiritists, the practice of Spiritism meant approaching life through a study of the spirit world and its moral and spiritual principles. It provided a way to continue to enrich their understanding of the world during a time of advanced age.

Marriage and Its Problems

As we reviewed our memories of the women in the room, it became clear that most of the social attributes of the therapists and healers in the Project were quite similar to those of most women of our acquaintance in Puerto Rico. Those in the health professions had sought to raise their social status by acquiring education—without giving up their traditional roles as wives and mothers. Some had already suffered conflict in marriage, but that had not impeded either their professional activities as therapists, nurses, or doctors or their avocations as Spiritist healers. Although difficulty in marriage may be part of the package of disturbances that assists the decision to become either a healer or a health professional, these women are probably no more vulnerable to such problems than are other women in Puerto Rico.

We recalled a study of women in lower and middle socioeconomic classes that showed basically similar patterns in women's expectations of their roles as wives, regardless of social class (Muñoz Vásquez, 1979). Women who have achieved professional, and therefore middle class, status do not expect to behave differently in marriage to compensate for a career and its time burden. Whether or not they share in decision making, have any power over the financial resources of the household, or get their needed share of affection, opportunities for personal growth seem to depend upon the individual woman and her and her spouse's expectations of each other. Although the group of women described in this book are about equally divided between lower- and middle-class backgrounds (using education as the main criterion), they share common problems in reconciling their personal values and vocational achievements with the widely accepted value put on superlative motherhood. As we discussed this widespread dilemma, we recalled Christensen's comment that he was "struck" by the "universality of the squeeze women feel between the positive valences of work, education, family and social life. Cultural determinants make it difficult for these women to consider giving less to any of these parts of their lives" (1979:59).

Stories of difficulties in marriage are commonplace among these women healers.

> One young medical doctor recalled her marriage to a well-known radio announcer while attending medical school in the Dominican Republic. This angered her parents who ceased supporting her when she informed them some eight months after the event. On the couple's return to Puerto Rico, her husband had trouble earning a living and her small son was frequently ill. She

> felt severely over-burdened with all of the responsibilities of the care of the child and household, as well as carrying the greatest part of the financial burden of the family.

Another doctor, in order to avoid what she called a "double load" and great resentment toward her husband, moved in with her mother. A third physician reported that she divorced her husband because he would not share the financial burdens of the family—even though she said that, formerly, she "did not believe in divorce."

Some of the mental health workers gave similar accounts of difficulties with spouses, but as a group they seemed less troubled by burdens arising out of career demands. We noted that these demands were less extensive and somewhat less compelling and time consuming than those experienced by physicians. Almost half of the mental health professionals had not yet married at the time we talked with them, but several were betrothed or planned to marry in the near future. Many of those who were married reported that they had had difficulties with their husbands but were currently winning the struggle to juggle their domestic roles, jobs, and, for some, schooling for advanced degrees.

We sought out Della, a good example of someone who was juggling many roles successfully, according to her own assessment. She had been married for twenty-two years and had raised three children (then ages sixteen to nineteen). After working as a teacher for seven years, she had returned to the university to acquire higher degrees in special education and social work. Della continued to work as a teacher and also studied, even though her oldest child was then only four years old and her youngest still an infant. On meeting Della, one could not deny her sense of high energy, strength of character, and conviction. In describing her marriage, she related that her only significant problem was that she could not share her husband's intense involvement with Spiritism. Della came from a traditional Catholic family that disapproved of Spiritist beliefs and practices. But Della was the type of woman who vigorously came to grips with problems of all kinds. Her involvement with our project emerged from her desire to better understand and share her husband's belief in Spiritism.

Two other mental health workers who were divorced felt that they had suffered a great deal while married. They explained that they had "fallen into" relationships with "irresponsible" men. They were now successfully demonstrating their capacity to raise their children alone and manage their households without spouses.

Most of the Spiritists we saw in the conference room had been married for many years and felt fulfilled in having successfully reared a number of children. They were now being rewarded with grandchildren. However, when many of these women discussed their marriages, they bitterly joked about the ways in which their husbands had been irresponsible, especially in the early years. Their men had regularly disappeared for drinking bouts with carousing friends or lovers or had had relationships with women *por la izquierda* (on the side). Husbands were described not only as irresponsible but also as very jealous. They used their position as *jefe de familia* (head of the family) to curb the extrafamilial activities and enthusiasms of their wives.

> Rosa told us that she was twenty-five years old when she had her first experience of spirits and disturbing visions that rendered her "nervous and out of control," unable to function normally as housewife and mother. Her husband was told by an *Espiritista* that she must be brought to a *centro* to be cured of spiritual problems. Rosa was "ordered" to set up a *mesa* (table) at which to work spiritually. Although after three months she was much better, her husband opposed her spiritual work until many years later, after she suffered numerous emotional and physical problems that she reported were caused by his drinking and philandering and her intense rage and jealousy.

The painful realities of married life seemed to us somewhat more important in the life stories of the older Spiritist healers than in the stories of the younger professional women or in those of the few Spiritist healers who had professional careers. Doña Margarita, still involved in her *lucha* (struggle) with her husband after thirty-two years, told us, "I have suffered a great deal because my husband is a pessimist, authoritarian, and *machista*. I am a 'live wire,' but he is very withdrawn and negative. This has caused much frustration and anxiety, so that I suffer from being anxious and from nervousness. We don't fit together."

In the same vein Doña Eulalia explained to us one evening that most of her problems stemmed from the fact that her husband had had a lover for twenty-two years. Although he always returned home and gave her sufficient money to pay the household bills, his infidelity caused her even more pain because she possessed the "faculty" to "see exactly what they were doing."

Both Doña Margarita and Doña Eulalia had been married for over thirty years and had never seriously considered divorce. This illustrates the extent to which a woman's self-concept and self-esteem are commonly bound up with spouse and mother roles. It seemed to us as we discussed the matter that not only is the suffering that accompanies prolonged marital difficulties expected in the truly feminine life but the dignity of being a "good" woman who suffers for the sake of her family definitely enhances feminine self-esteem. This unfortunate paradox appears to be directly related to illness and emotional distress, both of which are linked to experiences such as those mentioned previously in women's accounts of married life.

Early Lives

We often noted that particular family situations seemed to have had special consequences for women who became healers. Project participants frequently told us that their families modeled a special pattern of reaction to illness episodes. For these women, early family life consisted of learning specific religious philosophies and practices and relating these ideologies to the development of a caring attitude. Still another important aspect of their early family lives was the degree to which their mothers had fostered a desire to achieve professional status or similar social distinctions.

Doctors' Early Lives

The medical doctors we observed in the conference room had not told us very much about their early motivations to attend medical school. However, two of them recalled that their parents seemed to push them into a career in medicine. However, all of the young doctors said that the desire to become a doctor began in early childhood. Milagros recalled: It was always my fascination. Always when I entered a hospital, I became very excited." María told us: "In my family there was a theme of wanting to cure. My grandmother and mother prepared home remedies (*remedios caseros*) when someone became ill."

Although among the families of these young physicians only two sets of parents had achieved professional status themselves (the mothers were teachers), all of the women physicians were educated in private schools, which is the path to higher education and middle-class status in Puerto Rico. With one exception, parents of these women were recalled as having high expectations for them that were inevitably fulfilled.

One of the most important aspects of doctors' early lives was the early introduction and personal integration of a religious philosophy that espoused a firm sense of good and evil (Rodriguez Cortes, 1986–1987). All of these women said they considered themselves to be Catholics (having been baptized), most were educated by Catholic nuns during their primary school years, and a few attended mass with some regularity. Two were also influenced by significant others involved with Spiritist practices. All of them said that they possessed definite concepts of "good" and "evil." In their words, "good" means: "To help in all you can (other persons)," "something eternal that exists inside the person," "not to harm or hurt the feelings of anyone," "to be happy and right with God." "Evil" means: "To desire someone harm," "evil is the devil." All of the physicians said they believed in heaven and hell, or at the least in the survival of the soul after the death of the physical body. They especially seemed to believe that each life is predestined, that "the future of a person is already determined."

We could not help commenting (to each other) that all of these beliefs pointed to a well-defined morality focused on interpersonal relationships. In fact, there seems to be a special type of femininity that is the base upon which women's self-esteem rests in Puerto Rico. Women are "good" directly in relation to their concern for others; their self-identity works from the inside out, as Landy noted long ago (1959). Their major point of reference is their inner feelings toward significant others. We observed that the healers identified all the persons who sought them out as significant others, an unlimited extension of this moral pattern.

Mental Health Workers' Early Lives

We were told by the mental health professionals that early in their lives close relatives had experienced chronic illness. The mental health workers had also suffered their own, often unusual, bouts with illness during childhood. Elsa said:

> My mother always suffered from *nervios* [emotional distress]. She is now more stable than ever. But when I was in middle school my mother suffered a great deal. She was in psychiatric treatment and became crazy. On my father's side there's also some crazy people. My father's sister never left the mental hospital. There is an uncle, my father's brother, who hung himself. My father and we three [she and her sisters] existed in a different world.

Other women recalled similar experiences, such as a younger brother with Down's syndrome, a brother who was mentally retarded as the result of an accident, parents who drank too much and quarreled, and parents severely stressed by children with chronic mental illnesses. Given the deep significance of extended family ties for everyone in Puerto Rico, particularly as a supportive network, the illness of an aunt, uncle, cousin, or grandparent can lead to almost as much stress and upset as that of a parent. We observed that for mental health workers the choice of a "helping" profession seemed to be rooted in an acute sense of morality, as it was for the women doctors, and in their feeling that to be really "good" one had to help others. But we were also repeatedly made aware of how their own illnesses as children seemed to have influenced their personal philosophies. Mental health professionals had suffered as children from various ailments: a chronic heart ailment; loss of an ovary when thirteen years old due to a benign tumor (along with feared cancer); asthma; severe allergies, headaches, and tachycardia. Some reported on the intense distress they felt when their fathers left the family during their early childhood; most expressed an acute sense of abandonment and painful memories of mothers who were often troubled and ill.

> Nelda's father died when she was born. She recalled, "I don't know what he died from, but he freaked out when I was born because he was not able to deal with that." Although her mother remarried and had four more children, Nelda was raised by her aunt and grandmother "for economic reasons." They were deeply involved with the Pentecostal religion. She, too, believed in that religion "very much" until she was sixteen years old and married. At thirty-three, after a difficult divorce, she returned to the Pentecostal church because she felt she needed to seek spiritual help.

I reflected on the idea that although Nelda's experience seemed extreme in terms of the direct relation between her troubled life and her religious involvement, one also had to take into account her deep distress over being abandoned by both parents. Hector and I were both surprised to find that over half of the mental health workers said they felt emotionally distanced from their mothers because of their deaths or mental illness or because they were physically incapacitated.

> Alba felt that she had "never had her own life." Her mother suffered from *nervios* and was an alcoholic. Alba spent her life trying to hide her mother's alcoholism from the world until her mother began to walk around the town drunk. Despite Alba's extreme frustration and distress, her sisters left the task of caring for her mother to her because she had not married. Alba said her mother's problems stemmed from conflict with her father, whom Alba admired for his knowledge and liberal political views.

We had been told that a number of mothers of mental health professionals, abandoned by their husbands, sent their daughters to be raised by grandmothers or aunts. Although we knew that this was a common pattern in Puerto Rico, these women were left with intense feelings of abandonment. Several others said they were still angry that their mothers favored a sibling over them. One woman said she was the *patito feo* (ugly duckling) of her family; she argued a great deal with the sister her mother seemed to prefer.

Only a few women spoke of their early relationships with their mothers as having been satisfactory but resented being "overprotected" and not permitted to experience the freedom of their teenage years. Moreover, these overprotective mothers were recalled to have become intensely critical of their daughters in later years, severely affecting their daughters' sense of self-worth.

> Cecilia, a mental health worker, reported feeling "overprotected" as a child. She said she felt trapped and "put down" by her mother. Her mother continually alleged that Cecilia did not have the capacity to assist her with their farm. She reported that her feelings of low self-worth persisted, making her subject to

bouts of depression. She related this situation to current frustrations over not having found a suitable mate—at thirty years old.

Again we commented on how mothering (or feeling its lack) is associated with becoming a healer. There is a widespread cultural expectation that superlative mothering is the God-given right of all children. We also noted that the special emphasis on solidarity of women within a family may be a response to the pain of subservience and degradation. Therefore, failing to relate intimately and positively with one's mother, although difficult the world over, may be especially distressing to Puerto Rican women.

Spiritists' Early Lives

Those Spiritist healers who spoke to us about difficulties with their mothers or loss of their mothers were even more explicit than the mental health professionals about the distress this caused. As will be detailed later, much of their spiritual development seemed focused on recovering their mothers.

Most of the Spiritist healers (all but three of thirty-five) came from poor families and had had to work at unskilled jobs in order to support their children, younger siblings, or adopted children. Yet by the time we met them, they all seemed to have achieved some middle-class comforts as well as feelings of security—despite much illness, failed marriages and divorces for some, and many years of unhappiness for the majority.

However, a few Spiritist healers' mothers were remembered as having strong convictions on behalf of their daughters' futures. Evelyn recalled:

> I remember that my mother said, "For Evelyn, if God help me, I want her to be a teacher." My sisters had only gone to the second grade. But I continued growing and thinking about my mother's words. I went to school, and when I was going to go to second grade, my mother found a friend in town and this friend promised that if mother sent me to town she would help me out. And so that's what my mother did. She sent me every Sunday and I came home on Fridays and in this way this woman sent me to school. In order to go to school in the country, you had to cross large farms that looked like forests. There were no roads. But one day something happened. I don't know what. I know that my mother collected everything and came to town. She cried the whole way! She found a room and we got settled there. She began work as a cook, and my father worked as a carpenter. He earned only one dollar per day. But we improved because we all helped, and my little sister was able to go to school, too. My older sisters married, and the younger ones continued studying. When I was in fourth grade, I collected all the children in the barrio, and we played school. I was always the teacher.

Evelyn graduated from eighth grade in 1931. But it was twenty-six years before she was able to fulfill her dream of becoming a teacher, after evening classes were offered in her community. She finally graduated with honors from high school in 1960 and two years later obtained a teaching certificate from a normal school. Within a short time, Evelyn went from the job she held for eighteen years, cleaning the town buildings, to teaching school, from which she retired after sixteen years. She remembers a particular spirit revelation in which she saw herself giving classes, and the spirits told her she would be both a spiritual and "material" teacher. She said that her spirit guides provided the support she needed to achieve her mother's dream, and she considered the obstacles she faced as "trials" (*pruebas*) that simply had to be endured.

Although we felt that Evelyn's perseverance represented the extreme of a pattern of overcoming obstacles to achieve "materially," that is, to obtain a social goal, many of the Spiritist healers showed incredible fortitude in overcoming obstacles to achieve personal ends they had come to cherish.

It is significant that almost all of the Spiritist healers who did achieve a profession were either nurses or school teachers. We observed that their choices were bound in part by social convention. However, these choices reflected attitudes that were shaped in childhood about the high value of being a "helping" person.

Illness in early life seemed especially important for the Spiritist healers, because it frequently began a long involvement with spirit phenomena. In contrast to the doctors and therapists, many more Spiritist healers reported suffering life-threatening illnesses as children. When only seven years old, Milagros contracted "influenza." She recalled

> a great epidemic, where people died vomiting blood. There were no antibiotics or sufficient personnel in the hospitals to take care of them. The sick were attended to in the homes of families where up to sixteen people were ill. I got it lightly, and the only thing that sustained me was a glass of water. The water was put there by my mother, and the glass filled with *burbujas* of color. I didn't have to eat because the water had food in it!

From that time on, Milagros felt that she was "conscious of spiritual radiations."

We discussed the notion that Milagros had a certain mind-set about miraculous experiences. From birth she felt that she carried "a prediction of personal doom." She was told that she was a child who "cried in the womb three times" when her mother had carried her seven months. This is a belief that the baby will become a *persona agraciada* (especially lucky, blessed) but also may die.[1] Milagros felt that she had actually escaped her fate: she was a fat, healthy child at two years, because of her mother's spiritual powers and personal fortitude and despite her father's having abandoned them. As a result of the latter circumstance, her mother had to work as a servant and use her breast milk for children other than her own daughter.

We were told that most of the mothers of the Spiritist healers, as in the case of Milagros, believed in or practiced Spiritism; in a few cases, a grandmother or other relative had influenced the healer. Belief and practice ran in families and was passed on through women. Because the health of the family is considered to be the responsibility of the mother, many of these women had extensive knowledge of healing herbs and home remedies. This is no longer common among women who are fifty years old or younger because of the much greater availability of and belief in biomedical health care. However, primary responsibility for family health is still considered a vital part of the maternal role. We wondered whether this was associated with the fact that most Spiritist healers recalled suffering greatly over a sibling's illness or death.

> Lucita recalled her anguish when one of her brothers was ill. Even though she was still a small child, the strength of her religious attitude toward illness was illustrated by her response: she seized the Bible and began to read. Her brother became considerably better by the time she finished reading and got well. Later, when she was fourteen years old, she herself became sick at school. She "had heard people speak of the Rosicrucians, who were doctors of space." She asked these doctors if they could cure her, and that night she felt that some doctors had come to her room and cured her. She felt their presence. This proved that "doctors of space exist."

Emma vividly recalled the death of her twenty-two-year-old sister who suffered from tuberculosis and whom she loved as a mother. Emma was nine years old at the time. It was at this point that she began to be interested in Spiritism. Although baptized in the Catholic Church and schooled at a Catholic school, Emma had been taken to Spiritist centers by another sister and by her mother. After the tragedy, a medium brought the spirit of her recently departed sister to a session. The spirit predicted that all the brothers and sisters would "follow the same path," leaving only one to take care of their mother. Emma became extremely fearful that she, too, would die. Years later the prophecy was fulfilled, and only she remained. Through Spiritism, she said, she learned to understand and accept what she interpreted as a "spiritual debt" that her family had to pay.

Most of the Spiritists (as well as the doctors and therapists) told us that the Catholic Church did not provide satisfying answers to their questions about the personal tragedies they experienced or reasons for the distress they had to endure. Laura said, "I had a feeling for Catholicism, but although I went to church, I did not learn very much. It didn't give me much understanding."

She related that she was left an orphan at four years of age and was forced to go to church by her adoptive family. She associated much of their rigidity and conservatism with Catholicism and felt that the priests were immoral and played around with women. Laura lamented, "I didn't have a childhood." In her first experience with spirits at the age of ten, Laura saw the head of a man with long hair, cut off from his body and mounted on a zinc panel. This took place in the patio of her home and was confirmed by a neighbor.[2] She said she knew that her biological mother was a Spiritist, and she was "born with *facultades* [powers] to see into the spirit world."

We reflected upon the idea that by becoming a healer Laura established a connection with the mother she had scarcely known. However, it also kept alive memories of the cruel mother who reared her.

Observations

Mothers are especially sacred figures in Puerto Rico. The source of their sanctity is symbolized in the image of the Virgin, during and after the death of her Son. Mothers are supposed to sacrifice everything for their children, including their own happiness. Moreover, they are expected to derive their happiness from their offspring. Although many mothers in Puerto Rico seem actually to live up to the ideal, perhaps to a greater extent than mothers elsewhere (this would be extremely difficult to measure), they are also exquisitely human. But mothers can and do have negative effects on their children, especially on their daughters (Chodorow, 1978). The social and economic circumstances of Puerto Rican womanhood conspire to unbalance what I believe is a genuine desire to mother in an ideal way. During our project, I often had the thought that women most often become healers to reconnect with, or become, their lost mothers. When a daughter perceives herself as having been abandoned, or actually has been, the need for reparation is especially intense, given the cultural emphasis on the lifelong importance of mother-daughter relationships. As an example of this idea, Lolita, a Spiritist healer who perceived herself abandoned by her mother, candidly described how her first experience with a spirit was a reaction to abuse by her mother.

> When I was eight years old my mother mistreated me. I was the scapegoat of the family. After my mother hit me, I went to bed to cry. An old man with red hair came and sat on the bed and told me his name. He gave me the following message: "You will go with your father wherever he is going on Friday." I told the man that my mother had mistreated me. Then I felt much better and calmer. Later, I told my father what happened, and he went to a closet and found a picture of his father. This was the same old man I had seen and heard in my vision!

Lolita's deceased grandfather had been a well-known Spiritist healer. She was then taken to Spiritist sessions by her father and maternal grandmother. Although beset by illness most of her life (she underwent twenty-one operations) and having had great difficulty bearing children, she told us that her Spiritist beliefs and practices had sustained her for fifty years.

Notes

1. Such beliefs are no longer widespread, but they connote a religious philosophy often referred to indiscriminately as "fatalism." A more accurate explanation is that life was so uncertain in Puerto Rico until World War II, because of extreme impoverishment and poor health, that it was believed that life and death were controlled by forces much greater than one's personal efforts. Such matters were in the hands of God.

2. Even if we view this vision as a projection of her anger toward a strict stepfather and six rowdy stepbrothers, who made her life miserable, its impact as a painful memory is evident.

3

Callings: Healers' Initiatory Experiences

Only human beings guide their behavior by a knowledge of what happened before they were born and a premonition of what may happen after they are dead. Thus only human beings find their way by a light that illumines the patch of ground they stand on.

—Peter and Jean Medawar, *The Life Science*

Accounts of traditional healers in many societies focus on the importance of their dealings with the forces of darkness, symbols of all that is negative and evil. Events leading to their initiations as healers commonly include torturous battles and conquests of ubiquitous evil beings (Wallace, 1966; Eliade, 1964). But most accounts of healer initiations are about men, such as Peters' (1981) book on a Nepalese shaman. There are some descriptions of women's initiations into a healer role (Jones, 1966; Snow, 1977; Leacock and Leacock, 1975; Russell, 1984; Kendall, 1985; McClain, 1989), but many lack detail and depth on the psychology of initiation or, most important, on what the women themselves experience, as opposed to prescribed experiential patterns. Initiation as a process or as a stage of psychological development is not formally celebrated by mental health professionals or medical doctors, nor is it thought of as requisite to becoming a psychological or medical healer. Therefore, this chapter mostly describes the initiatory experiences of Spiritist healers. However, I describe the informal initiations of mental health professionals and medical doctors where permitted by our observations.

Initiations of shamans commonly center on how the fledgling healer overcomes threats of world destruction and acquires special powers and knowledge on behalf of humankind. In partial contrast to the healer initiations of men, those of women seem more focused on overcoming intimate, inner evils, personified as evil spirits that invade and possess the initiate's body. Dealing with one's own suffering becomes central to the challenge of developing powers to heal others. Thus inward threats are highly significant to women as healers, even more so than destruction and evil emanating from the world outside.

This gender difference is reflected in the idealized patterns of women's versus men's lives in Puerto Rico. The well-known dichotomy of a woman's place being in the home and a man's being "in the streets" is integral to thinking about male and female roles and spheres of influence. Although men become healers of all types, intimacy and inner life is largely given over to women. Thus men as Spiritist healers (although there are fewer of them than women) are usually leaders and organizers of *centros*, while women carry out most of the healing work by taking spirits into their bodies. In a parallel way, men as medical doctors and mental health professionals hold many more of the leadership and administrative positions, while women more often work in the trenches carrying out the "scut work," the detailed tedium of everyday patient care.

As Hector and I looked around the seminar room, we again confirmed our observation that whether spirit healers, psychotherapists or medical doctors, women as healers are involved in a continual process of development, both personally and as healers—actually one and the same process. We had been told about the first initiatory experiences of the *Espiritistas*, described as awakenings of consciousness to spirits, which most frequently begin during childhood or adolescence. This first stage of initiation was described by eight of thirteen male Spiritist healers in the project and by twenty-two of the thirty-five female Spiritists as occurring early in life. But they also told us that there is a point in time when a decision is taken to "work" at development of the healing faculties. Most often, this decision is immediately preceded by a personal crisis, usually serious illness. The Spiritists described their initiations into healer roles as personal transformations, while the psychotherapists and medical doctors spoke of the process of becoming healers more simply, as the appropriate steps in the development of a career plan. Health professionals only occasionally examined the implications of their feelings about what they had experienced prior to or in becoming healers, when we prompted the exploration.

Antecedents to Becoming a Healer: The Spiritist Experience

Nine of the thirty-five Spiritist healers recalled seeing spirits when very young, between the ages of five and eight years; thirteen others first saw or heard spirits when ten to eighteen years old; six when young adults; and the rest in middle age. All of the healers remembered the experience as a vivid, intense event, triggered in a number of cases by worry about death, or the actual death, of a loved person. Even as young children, the Spiritists could identify these spirits as parents, grandparents, aunts, uncles, or siblings who "had passed over." Other recollections of spirits were of friendly beings, ranging from saints to one's own spirit in a former life. Illness or emotional distress was an important aspect of a first experience with spirits. In one case, a child, whose mother abused her, was comforted by her grandfather's spirit. Spirits were occasionally reported to have bothered healers as children, but most experiences were positive in that the spirits gave help or emotional support in times of crisis.

Some parents of healers accepted their child's experience of spirits as helpful, while others seemed to ignore it. In two cases where parents were fervent Catholics, healers recalled that spirit experiences were interpreted as emotional disturbances in the child. However, none of the parents are remembered to have punished their children or responded negatively.

Half of the Spiritists said that one or both parents, or grandparents, practiced as healers or believers. Others recalled being taken to *centros* where relatives presided or worked. Thus expectations about spirit experiences developed within a familial context of belief. What seemed important to us as observers was that spirits rather than living beings offered support at times of remembered great need. Certainly these healers share a special quality, an inner capacity to work through distressing problems defined as crises. In many this ability began in childhood with spirit experiences, while others acquired it as the result of an adult crisis, usually an experience of life-threatening illness in themselves, their parents, or their children. The process of "development of faculties" to become a medium appeared to us to be thought of as a learned way to "switch on" feelings of well-being through contact with guide spirits (*guías*) identified as protectors. The initial experience of a *guía* spirit in the development process appears to be a direct transfer of positive affect associated with childhood experiences. It transcends distress caused by the disappearance through death of a beloved person or by feelings of helplessness or vulnerability.

Initiatory Illnesses

Having heard the healers' stories, we knew that the types of illness associated with initiatory experiences vary but generally include both physical and emotional complaints. We reflected that the healers could have, and have been considered by some to suffer from, psychiatric illness. However, most of these women had never received mental health care or been diagnosed as mentally ill, with two exceptions. One Spiritist had been hospitalized for psychiatric illness several times before she was forty years old, and another has received ambulatory psychiatric care over the last 15 years. After describing initiatory illness experiences, I will discuss our speculations whether most of the healers can be thought to have suffered undiagnosed episodes of mental illness and whether we could say that they were "cured" by becoming healers.

Anna was twenty-two years old when the spirits literally "threw her to the floor." Her family described these as "convulsive attacks" that did not appear to be epilepsy. As a result, Anna began to frequent Spiritist *centros* and often "transformed into other people." She said she actually took on the personalities of other people. This made her afraid that "she would do some harm." She prayed to these same spirits, but nothing happened. After a while, she stopped going to the *centros* because she "did not like the way they worked."[1]

Later, Anna again took the healer role in a *centro* in Puerto Rico, one that conformed more to Kardecian practice. She was observed having the same sort of "convulsive attacks," but they did not lead to possession by spirit beings. During these attacks, the other mediums merely left her alone unless she became aggressive, which sometimes occurred, and then they would exert some control over her through their *guías*. At other times, she became possessed in the accepted way; spirits spoke through her with "great clarity."[2]

Hector and I discussed the fact that the advent of a severe illness as the route to initiation into the healer role has been described for a great many cultures (Wallace, 1966; Lewis, 1971). Strikingly similar experiences are reported across societies. Evelyn's account, which will be presented next, has all of the "classic" features, particularly with regard to how her illness deteriorated into a deathlike state. She reports that she felt as if she were actually dead. She and others recalled that after such an experience, recovery was often slow, but upon recovering, the events of the illness took on meaning as the first stage of a personal transformation. In our view, this is achieved through a process of cognitive and emotional restructuring of self in both inner and outer worlds. The transformed person remembers gradually beginning to feel different and acquires a much greater sense of inner peace and well-being, which she works to maintain. We recalled how the new healer, as an apprentice, said she embarked upon her "life mission" aimed at helping others, who like herself continued to suffer. She also continued to transform personally as an integral part of her healing work; she literally became a "wounded" healer, continually healing her own illness as she helped others.

Evelyn recalled:

I began to feel weak, lost weight, my mind was chaotic, I was irritable, the economic situation was terrible, and I began to look for work. But I didn't feel good, and because I depended on public welfare, one wasn't cared for well when you went to a doctor. At that time I went to church, took communion, confessed, and prayed to God for my health and also for my dead mother. Each day I felt worse. When I walked, I felt like I walked on air. My husband decided to take me to the hospital and some *padrinos* (godparents) found someone who could get me a bed and they left me for twenty days, but nothing happened. I came home the same. I got a "mania" for water. I couldn't be quiet; all day, agitated.

I couldn't do anything. I sat. A friend told me, "You should go to an *Espiritista* because it looks like you have something." I answered her: "I don't believe in that. The spirit is the blood, and after a person dies it doesn't leave."

They gave me tap-water baths, sea baths, well baths. They gave me many remedies and dealt with me, but it seemed that nothing helped because I lacked faith. I was failing, and then I decided to go to the *centros*, but I doubted too much. One day the girl who had told me to go to an *Espiritista* appeared at my house . . . and according to what she later told me, this day I looked pale, but she didn't say anything to avoid scaring me. The only thing she said was, "You are still drinking water." I remember that when she told me that, I couldn't avoid it, but a very loud shout came out of me of which I was aware, but nothing more. I didn't know anything more about the world.

Well, they took me to an *Espiritista*, but I was so *rabiosa* (wild), *riendome* (laughing) at these things; well, I believed that they had separated my body from my spirit and left me accompanied by some spirit. It was like I had faculties and was so hardened (*endurecida*). Perhaps because of this I had to suffer that very bitter experience. I didn't know where I was. In my ear I heard someone who said to me: "Look, now you are with me. You don't have a body because look where your body is." He showed me the living room of my house. I didn't see anything, I didn't see people in the house; that is, my body didn't sense anything—only a gray coffin (*un ataúd de gris*) with my body inside, and it [the voice] was repeating many times: "Now you know that spirits exist. Look where your body is in that box. Do you see?" Repeated many times, but at that moment I saw nothing. I wasn't on the earth. I don't know where I was, nor who spoke to me. I didn't have a body—nothing, nothing. In a moment, I felt like the blood was circulating and my feet were feeling the ground, but I tried to open my eyes and couldn't. At that moment, with my eyes closed, I saw a tall black woman with a dress woven of a very thick thread, but she was smiling (I guess this would be my *madama* [spirit image of a woman obeah healer; obeah is a Caribbean folk religion]). But I felt so afraid when she saw my surprise, and in that moment I opened my eyes.

It hadn't occurred to anyone to move me or take me to the hospital. I heard someone say, "She is dead because she doesn't have any blood." "Look how white her eyes are; if she's alive she looks like a cadaver." When I heard these words, I jumped up. I couldn't walk. I tell you my whole body shook with the shake of cold death. I shook to my very eyes. I left running, fleeing, went through the kitchen, and I went in back of the house, and there I leaned against the wall trembling, tired, fleeing those people, because I believed I was really dead because of such a long period that I lost. But someone saw me and took me to bed; they rubbed *alcoholado* (perfumed alcohol) on me. Then they sent for my husband, who was working for a man who knew Spiritism. And he began to cope with me and said, "Today this woman has developed her faculties; I see this house always full of people, because I see her working with many people."

After resting in bed for two weeks, "praying for understanding," Evelyn was taken to a *centro*, and an *Espiritista* told her: "You have faculties.

Everything that has happened to you is spiritual, and you have to work." Evelyn continued to have many "revelations" that directed her in her new "work," such as the instruction to prepare a *centro* in her home. She also dreamed that she had died and had seen people with halos. She said that she continued to get better as she worked at *la obra* (healing work). At some point, she returned to the hospital for tests, which were all "negative."

We found it interesting that Evelyn never mentioned if or how she had been diagnosed by doctors. It is likely that they told her something about her condition, but that fact seemed almost irrelevant because she was so convinced that the cause and condition were spiritual in nature.

We wondered about the role of an initiatory illness such as this, because it is so complex and not well understood. In the accounts of the Spiritist healers, the important elements are the images of death invoked, the experience of the conscious self leaving the body and yet able to observe it from a distance, and the difficulty of returning from a state of nonbeing to the mundane, familiar world. These experiences are well documented by numerous analysts of "altered states of consciousness," such as Ludwig (1969). First perceptions of separation of the self-conscious center of being from the body always cause emotional upheavals. A strong emotional impact occurs because familiar landmarks of adaptive feeling and thinking lose their meanings. The intimate and common ground of assumptions about the world, such as the internal marking of the passage of time, is violently shaken. A usual landscape of perception becomes distorted and chaotic. We had observed how in Spiritism, as in religious healing in many societies, this extreme alteration in everyday consciousness is interpreted as a death/rebirth experience of a special kind. A redefined sense of self emerges from the experience, and the initiate becomes possessed with a compelling dedication to a new way of actualizing life through spirit work and healing.

Normal or Abnormal?

When we reviewed Evelyn's narrative of her initiatory illness with regard to the extensive alterations in consciousness she experienced, certain features seemed quite specific to Spiritism and also to other Latin healing traditions. The deathlike state to which she attributed the separation of conscious awareness from her body, the loss of her sense of being embodied, and the simultaneous paralysis of her sense of time did not constitute a "death" conceived of as the end of bodily and mental sensations but rather a "passing over" into a spirit state of being. We were told by the Spiritists that this experience acts as a connection to the cosmos, of which the visible world is only a small portion. To be able to alter consciousness and enter this experience in a controlled way is to enter a state of transcendence while still

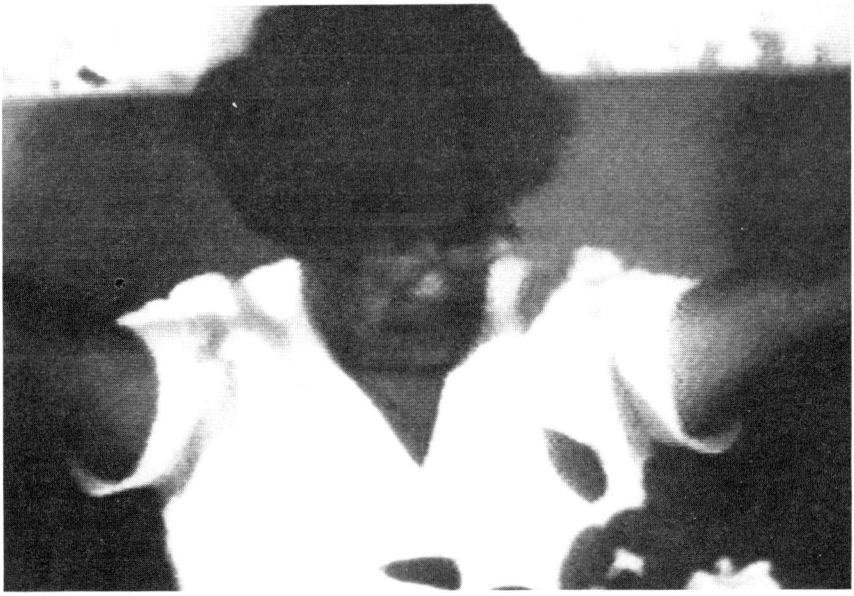

While opening a session, a *centro* president is possessed by her spirit guide.

alive—and be able to do so repetitively. (See also Garrison, 1979; Nuñez, 1987.)

We thought about how Spiritist mediums learn how to enter the nonliving world of spirits, the world of those who have "crossed over." This is done at will (although it may occur involuntarily at the beginning of development and during crises). Mediums initially experience a state of chaos and even of fear but gradually are able to exert more and more control over their "passing over" into the spirit world, which is done only when deemed ritually appropriate. We knew from the mediums' stories that altering consciousness can have both adaptive and maladaptive consequences for the healers themselves. In our opinion, it is control over altering one's state of conciousness that makes the crucial difference when judging whether it is psychopathological. According to Wintrob and Pattison (1981), hallucinations and delusions are pathological when they lead to maladaptive rather than to adaptive behavior.

In Spiritism visions are used in the service of healing others—this is both the goal of altering consciousness and its effect—so we judged it to be adaptive behavior. We observed and recorded two main types of consciousness-altering states entered into by Spiritists during their ritual healing sessions. The principal one is parallel to that defined as "possession-trance" by Bourguignon (1975), because Spiritists say that a spirit being (whether good or bad) comes into the body of the healer. They say that they "lend" their bodies to the spirits to allow them to speak to their clients as the spirits request. When first "developing faculties," spirits come into a novitiate's body unbidden, causing great disturbances, such as trembling and thrashing about, as well as feelings of discomfort and faintness. After practicing mediumship for a number of years, adepts testify that they are affected very little when their own spirit guides come into their bodies. I have watched them tremble only slightly; their voices change only a bit. They themselves report a feeling of a pleasant chill in their bodies and a gentle cool breeze over their heads and backs. These sensations are described as "refreshing currents," "my body feels lighter," "tranquility," and "well-being" (*saludable*). Only in rare cases, when a new *guía* presents itself, may the transition between states of consciousness be somewhat rougher. In contrast, possession by a "backward" *causa* (illness-causing) spirit is extremely difficult and almost always chaotic, even for very practiced mediums.

We noted that the second kind of alteration of everyday consciousness is also an integral part of the ritual session. This seems to be a variant both of the hypnotic state and of active daydreaming into which imagery comes (Singer, 1976). This state of consciousness does not seem to cause distress for most medium-healers and is often partly shared by clients and onlookers. As mediums describe it, it is essentially a meditative state, induced by repetitive praying followed by a quiet space in which they silently pray and "look inside." Mediums report that in their experiences the spirit world is usually visual but is sometimes auditory.

The ability to develop elaborate images of spirits on behalf of persons in distress and to understand the meanings of these imaged spirits is the hallmark of "developing faculties," according to our participants. This ability is described as a special kind of communication, a "seeing into" a superordinate spirit world through which the medium learns about the past-life conditions of the client or anyone seeking help. This way of "knowing" is reported to be most often acquired during the initiatory illness. It also seems to be potentially available to some healers from early childhood; for them this ability is reinforced during their initiatory illness.

We knew that the creation of an alternative, nonphysical world as part of one's personal sphere of action is considered pathological by many psychiatrists. But the imagery of schizophrenics seems far less elaborate than that of the medium-healers and does not conform to agreed-upon definitions. As pointed out by Jerome Singer (1976), the hallucinations and delusions of schizophrenics act to further isolate them from human contact; persons having psychotic symptoms suffer a general, pervasive disturbance in their ability to relate to others. The spirit imagery of Spiritist healers has a precisely opposite effect; it functions to enhance interpersonal relating. Most important for the healer is the part it plays in her special therapeutic role by linking

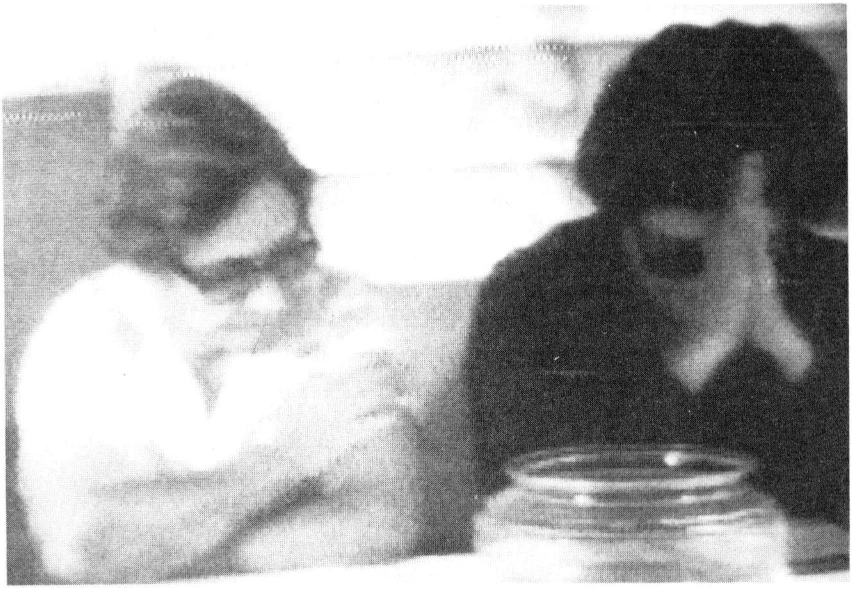

At a *centro* session, a medium describes a *videncia* about a client to a companion medium.

her to her patient and connecting both healer and patient to a spiritual universe ordered by humanistic, moral principles. We knew that the Spiritist healers act as channels, allowing distressed persons to reexperience human-spirit relationships from previous incarnations in order to understand and solve current problems and ills. By confronting these problems, believed to have come from previous incarnations, healers report that both they and their clients mutually participate in a sacred process of spiritual evolution as part of the Holy Spirit's plan to create an ideal world based on high moral sentiments and peace.

Communications with and from the spirit world are intended to be confined to ritual occasions. One reason Spiritist healers give for preferring to work as part of a team is that they can support one another in dealing with the more distressing, dangerous elements of the spirit realm. We reflected upon the view that this is normal for a society like Puerto Rico where large numbers of people believe in the effectiveness of supportive action in groups—especially when confronted with problems or danger. Although possession-trance and spirits speaking in a bizarre way may look "crazy" to an outsider, they seem entirely appropriate in Puerto Rico (and also elsewhere) within an agreed-upon ritual context. Therefore Spiritist possession-trance cannot be said to even mimic psychotic behavior, if the latter is defined as "confused thinking" or "inappropriate communication."

In the case of one Spiritist healer (out of the thirty-five in this group) who suffers psychiatrically diagnosed psychotic episodes and intermittent hospitalizations, we saw that the episodes clearly interfered with her healing activities and prevented her from working with spirits. My impression is that spirit healing is so onerous, so physically and psychologically demanding, that a healer must enjoy an above-average level of psychological well-being to carry out weekly ritual practices. Contrary to many medical and psychological definitions of well-being, this does not mean being completely free of illness or from inner or outer conflict. Rather, it means ideally being able to continually cope with personal adversity without breakdown into physical or mental illness. Further, it appears that the initiatory illness becomes meaningful to the new healer as a recognition that she can cope with serious, even life-threatening, difficulty. Subsequent problems and illness appear to be manageable and relatively insignificant compared to this first traumatic event. It is possible that becoming a Spiritist healer has the adaptive consequence of preventing mental illness in some persons who are predisposed to it by other factors, but it would be impossible for ethical reasons to run double-blind studies to demonstrate this hypothesis.

Receiving the Guías

The initiatory illness and accompanying ability to alter consciousness were reported to be only the beginning of the process of self-transformation. We received many descriptions of how the initial experience is later built upon by a continual process of receiving and relating with the spirits identified as guide-protectors. For example, Evelyn described a "tall, black woman" who had rather primitive clothing and was smiling. In her account of the experience, she identified this woman as her *madama*, a frequent initial spirit guide-protector of women healers.

The *guías* are the healer's spirit supports and helpers, both in her healing work and in her life. The more moral the healer's intentions and acts, the greater the likelihood that she will attract helpful spirit guides. The role of the principal *guía* in the healing session is to preside over the work. After possessing the healer at the beginning of the session, the guide-protector stands behind her, available to assist when ignorant, backward, illness-causing spirits get out of hand. This principal *guía* again presides at the close of the healing session. *Guías*, especially the main protector-spirits, are reported to confer the strength and determination that the healer-as-heroine must possess to carry out her life mission. The smile on the *madama* spirit's face shows her approval of Evelyn and her consent to support and protect her.

We discussed the fact that the *madama* spirit is an Afro-Caribbean obeah worker, a descendant of the West African pantheon. These gods and goddesses have the widespread reputation of being powerful as healers, sorceresses, and witches. To have such a spirit come to you as a personal guide-protector confers the possibility of that same power being available for spirit work, as well as being a personal resource. The description of the *guía*'s "woven dress" shows her to be a woman of rural background, lacking in sophistication but rich in contact with earthy things. Other prominent female spirit guides are gypsies or very old women (*ancianas*). One healer described her old woman as, "la *madre espiritual* (spiritual mother) who comes in moments of suffering." For three women in the group (and for several other mediums I have known), their principal *guía* is a mother or grandmother who died during their childhood. In the relatively rare cases where the main *guía* is a male spirit, we noted that the healer had had a particularly close relationship with her father or grandfather and often a difficult one with her mother.

We talked about how the ubiquity of strong feminine figures among principal *guías* is to be expected if we recall the pervasive ambivalent feelings women hold in relation to their mothers. The *madama guías*, as well as the gypsies and old women, all represent types of women who are marginal to ordinary society and have attributes that are feared by both men and women. They belong to a genre of female figures who are often seen as sorceresses and witches, attractive because of their underground power but also repulsive because of their perceived ability to turn power toward evil ends (Cixous and Clement, 1986). Observing through a psychological lens, one sees that these *guías* make possible a continued awareness of a negative feminine aspect of the self, a potential for cruelty as well as strength. Because the cultural ideal for Puerto Rican women—especially from a male perspective—is the passivity and goodness of the Virgin, the sorceress-witch appears as an unconscious, unacknowledged counterpoint in women's psyches. That the sorceress-witch probably exists in every woman is attested by the fact that although mother-daughter love is culturally exalted, actual relations between mothers and daughters are often anything but ideal. Women deeply resent the preference shown by their mothers to their brothers. This resentment is rarely voiced because there is no approved cultural context for its expression. Moreover, the dynamics of the so-called Electra triangle, in which mothers uncomfortably repel their latency-age (and older) daughters' attentions and coquetry toward their fathers, create still deeper chords of resentment and jealousy.

It is our understanding that beyond these usually masked conflicts is a subtle but pervasive problem in female identification, very much like that described by Eichenbaum and Orbach (1983a). Mothers' dependency needs and their basic sense of lack of entitlement, both as persons and as women, deeply affect their relationships with their daughters. Little girls learn early that mother is distressed and try to be what mother wants them to be. This means that they, too, must contain their own needs and never expect much satisfaction. This inner dynamic begins at the early age of five or six years. Women then grow up feeling fraudulent, because their mothers have set them up so that they do not expect nurturance when they are no longer small children. Thus daughters develop feelings that their own needs must eternally be subordinated to those of others if they are to be loved, especially by familiar males.

It is this lack of entitlement, the insistence that everyone must come before the woman and her concerns, that makes the healer role a repulsive one for Puerto Rican feminists. Because most of the *Espiritistas* are older than the health professionals, one can examine how their beliefs and practices work for or against this eternal dilemma. The life stories we heard revealed that the popular *madama* and other part-sorceress, part-witch *guías* express inner conflict over the fraudulent, unentitled feminine self but also represent a kind of resolution to that inner conflict. These *guías* are talked about as if they were eternally supportive and powerful, much like an inner wish for an ideal mother. It is noteworthy that the *madama* and old women *guías* have no hesitation in demanding gratification of their needs and desires. However, we were told that *guías* properly manifest only within a ritual context and not as conscious (or disruptive) forces in healers' everyday lives. Although we can appreciate *guías* as expressions of repressed or unavailable aspects of the healer's self, which is composed of many subpersonalities, they did not seem to us to be well-integrated into the Puerto Rican healer's psyche, even though fully acknowledged and more or less worshipped.

Eichenbaum and Orbach (1983a:96) describe how this inner dilemma manifests in their therapy with women. "All the women we have seen in therapy have come with problems and confusions about their sense of self because they did not embody enough of mother to allow them to separate. As this aspect of woman's psychology emerges in therapy, the wish to merge, to be closely connected to the therapist—as well as the anxiety this arouses—is a subtext running through the relationship."

Difficulties for women in acknowledging control and power and in feeling entitlement seemed at that time to be especially acute and severe in Puerto Rico, a Latin, male-oriented culture caught in turbulent crosscurrents of conflicting values composed of the traditional and the imported. Moreover, in a society (still) so tragically focused on cultural survival, the space within which to voice one's needs as a woman is sadly constricted.

Two mediums reported that God was their *guía principal*, although others frequently said that God and the saints were "too high" and "too involved or enlightened" to come to the table to assist in a medium's work. However, the mediums often said that everyone works through God or Jesus; it is He who ultimately heals. But it is interesting that the mediums who claim God as their main spirit guide have not developed the faculty "to speak," that is, they do not become possessed so that spirits can speak through them. Their *guías* do not then play the crucial role of protector-guide during the ritual healing sessions. I believe that this is an aberrant psychological relationship, quite different from the developed self-awareness of women who have *madamas* or spiritual mothers as their principal guides.

Although the principal spirit guide is most often a female spirit, most mediums have a *cuadro* (group, picture) of *guías* that includes both male and female spirits. Anna, for example, listed seven *guías*.

> (1) A doctor who helps her with "sick people" is "quite young, dark-skinned with dark hair. I saw him [just] this year"; (2) A nurse. "I saw her at the beginning of last year—young, strong, white [skinned]"; (3) "A girl about nine years old, she is a spirit with a great deal of light [who] gives me spiritual strength for problems. She gives me conformity [and] resignation to go forward"; (4) "A nun [who] gives orientation to confused persons." (This spirit is her aid in transmitting spiritual knowledge and speaking with spirits.); (5) An old woman, "the spiritual mother," described as her deceased grandmother; (6) A man dressed as St. Francis of Assisi who "symbolizes humility. He helps me when I am sad and desolate. He inspires me and gives me strength"; and (7) An Indian. "He is strong, large. He gives spiritual balm [blessing] and herbal prescriptions. He is the symbol of medicine."

Some healers described only two or three *guías*, others many more. Some said that they could not describe their *guías* because they had not yet developed the faculties to see them, although one woman saw her *guías* in dreams but had no waking visions of them. Those who were unable to see into the spirit world felt their *guías*' presence and "knew" when they were beside them. Some *guías* were quite exotic, such as a Tibetan Lama, whom the medium saw as an "older person with a long white beard." He helped her intellectually and in meditation with "studies" and "predictions." Several healers described an *indio* (American Indian), who is "strong, stands straight, and sets rules." Islamic and Chinese elderly men came as doctors. Children who had died came to help their healer-mothers, and priests were common as guides who brought peace and spiritual presence. Each *guía* acted upon the medium in a special way and could be said to symbolize a special attitude or characteristic that the healer found positive and with which she wanted to identify. In addition, a particular *guía* often helped with a particular "faculty," such as the power to transport one's own spirit to another place for the purpose of helping an ill person.

Guías came to mediums at various times during mediums' "development" (throughout their lifetimes) and could also leave, presumably because they were no longer needed. We speculated that in psychological terms *guías* could in time become irrelevant to current "spiritual" development. We observed a rough correlation between important life events and the appearance of a particular *guía*, which was also suggested by Pressel (1977). During the years of my acquaintance with many healers, I came to realize that the process of "development," including the appearance and disappearance of *guías*, was more complex than I had originally thought, made up of distressful as well as positive periods of emotion-laden experience that went beyond particular events. The individual psychologies behind the development process and how *guías* represent denied or feared personal attributes and attitudes will be discussed in Chapter 4.

I must note that several mediums refused to describe their *guías*. One said she couldn't "because I am now sick." When this particular medium began developing faculties, she had a *madama* who she said had since left. She implied that she was now undergoing a period of change and didn't know precisely who her new *guías* would be. Other healers who refused to describe their *guías* expressed the feeling that it was "something very personal." One woman felt that the information might be used "unscrupulously by another medium to mystify her identity."

I felt that this last comment signified distrust of the interviewer, but it also referred to the real fear that another medium might introduce harm if she knew the first healer's protector-guides. Although such suspicions were not expressed by the health professionals, they are important dangers of the Spiritist-healer role, especially when the spiritual powers of the healer are in the process of "development." These dangers and their associated vulnerabilities will be discussed more fully later. The attitude of suspiciousness is mentioned here in order to emphasize how important the *guías* are as basic elements in the construction of a new and continuing sense of self.

Developing Faculties

We observed that although many women who came to the table were told that they were developing faculties, not all were encouraged to do so. Healers said that some clients were too vulnerable. We speculated that the diagnosis of "in development" is based on a nonspecific set of complaints, in that the "condition" is thought of as an inevitable part of the sufferer's destiny; it always has a transcendent or enobling meaning. In addition, the illness of "development" is a sign that protector-spirits are near, giving it a positive value. As noted by other researchers (Rogler and Hollingshead, 1965), this positive or progressive view contrasts directly with the denigration frequently suffered by women who present complaints diagnosed by doctors as purely "psychosomatic" or as mental illness.

It has been widely reported in descriptions of Spiritist practices in New York (Garrison, 1977a, 1979; Harwood, 1977) that *guías* are propitiated by prayer, candle lighting, the wearing of special clothing, and the dedication of objects and promises on home altars. In Puerto Rico such practices exist but are considered both wrong and superstitious by those who believe in the "purer" (closer to Kardecian principles) practice of Spiritism. Although Puerto

Rican *Espiritistas* are involved with practices Kardec did not describe in his writings, most reject further incorporation of Afro-Caribbean religious ideas and practices. Although continuing syncretism with *Santería* (the Cuban saints' cult) occurs in Puerto Rico, we were told that an important reason to exclude these "lower" practices is their depersonalization of the *guías* into more or less standardized saint-god figures.

The personal *guías* that were described by Spiritist healers fell under certain types. *Guías* such as the *madama* or the *indio* seemed to represent universal, idealized patterns for personal action that took on specific, self-related meanings.[3] The identification of deceased relatives as *guías* further individualized the medium's *cuadro* (picture) of spirits, as did the descriptions of special clothing worn by the common *guías*; for example, the "young doctor who, when he comes to my side, I see his blue or white robe" or the soldier "dressed in yellow who doesn't like to be asked questions." Each *guía* is said to have a special personality that determines the direction of the relationship with a healer-medium; all spirits are thought of as teachers of the medium. We noted that the potential variation of types of *guías* and relationships with *guías* was enormously complex. It provided a picture of an unfolding autobiographical drama occurring somewhere in the three-dimensional space around the healer, during both her ritual sessions and her everyday activities (Koss, 1979).

An important aspect of the healer-*guía* relationship was the actual or promised emotional support *guías* provided, which could be more effective in times of emotional distress than the support offered by one's living relatives (Jerome Frank, personal communication). Like most living relations, *guías* also had their negative sides: they exacted obligatory behavior and sometimes even inflicted distress. This was more likely to occur when they first appeared to the not yet fully developed healer, as in Evelyn's case, which was described earlier. Many *guías* are not perfect beings and can occasionally be licentious and earthy in ways the healers themselves said were not socially acceptable. One gypsy *guía*, for example, made her healer "happy at parties." A developed medium told us, "I respect my *guías* because they take good care of me and my clients, but especially of me, myself. . . . I have promised to comply with my *guías* in order to have some peace in the universe."

We read Garrison's descriptions (1977a, 1979) of the *guías* as "part-selves" of the mediums. She observes that they "enact the 'superego functions.' . . . They also represent some 'ego functions' such as 'judgment' and 'intellectual processes.' They may, in addition, however, represent the 'libido' as, for example, when a *madama* or *conga* likes to 'talk frankly' about the pleasures of sex" (1979:432). Garrison makes a good case for the equivalence of Freudian psychoanalytic models of the self and Spiritist self-concepts. She equates *causa* spirits and the id, the ego and the *propio ser* (one's own spirit), and the guardian angel and most *guías* and the superego. But Hector and I decided that this parallelism only works for Spiritists if one believes that these basic psychic components of the self are not bounded by the skin. We concluded that a sense of the self as having boundaries appeared irrelevant for medium-healers.[4]

Psychological Aspects of Development as a Healer

Who then are *guías* in ethnopsychological (people's own) terms? If they are parts of the self, how is the self conceived by Spiritists? In my view, if we consider the "self" as a special kind of unity that provides both a sense of personal continuity with the universe and a sense of individuality in self-aware individuals, we get close to the notion of "spirit" according to Kardecian Spiritism. The idea of the spirit as integral to defining a human being resulted from Kardec's and his followers' reactions against the materialistic worldviews that emerged with the development of the study of science during the last half of the nineteenth century. Today Kardec (and many Spiritists) might say that the spirit incarnate is dependent upon the brain for its existence. But he said it can also exist without a physical envelope between incarnations and when it has come securely into the "light" and is no longer subject to being reincarnated.

The Spiritist self also depends upon a straightforward, simplified general life plan made up of values, morals, expectations, theories about how things should be and are, and appropriate goals and actions. The context for this life plan is a spirit world whose principles are clothed in symbolic, anthropomorphic garb. The *guías* are disembodied citizens of that world, idealized figures arranged in hierarchies of relative enlightenment to whom living beings have been related at some point in time. This world is relational, not fixed. Reading Kardec it seems clear that the opposite was clearly intended by him (and his many intellectual predecessors). The "self" of every spirit, whether incarnate or discarnate, gets its identity through participating in the master life plan. Each spirit understands how it fits into an evolving web of relationships aimed toward perfecting the spirit and participating in the all goodness and harmony of the universe. I view the beginning of "development" of the noviate healer as the means to uncover knowledge of these earlier relationships. To me the *guías* are condensed, imaginal representations of inner and outer relationships. This need for imaging the principles and structure of this world is crucial to a relational orientation to one's own experience of being, which is experienced at the same time as part of everything else in the universe.

Only in the sense I have described above can we call *guías* part-selves. In other words, for mediums (and others, especially women) interrelationship *is* being, but so also is individual integrity. This paradox is the basis of an essentially human process of individuation achieved through affiliation, described by many psychologists after Kardec. It was especially important, for example, to C. G. Jung, who was influenced by spiritualism. Jung (1969) believed that we are all part of a universal whole but also uniquely ourselves, especially after consciousness of self is achieved. As the famous biologist Theodosius Dobzhansky pointed out just before his death: "We are human beings because we are both self-aware and death aware" (1975:411).

In my view, Dobzhansky's observation perfectly captures the essence of the Spiritist process of "development of powers" as the way to acquire enlightenment. Consciousness of an overall life plan is essential to this process. Experiencing one's own death means confronting the end of the inner experience of one's individual integrity (one part of the paradox of the self) in order to experience its twin—oneness with a cosmic plan of life. In the Spiritist way of viewing the world, spirits are personified links between one's personal ("own") spirit and the "pure, Holy Spirit," which comprises the totality of the universal life plan. Once an individual is able to get through the fear of experiencing a halt in personal consciousness, she is then able to communicate with, and voluntarily experience the world of disembodied spirits. She then knows her own mortality but also her immortality—both interrelated aspects of the overall plan of life itself.

Receiving Women: Initiation of Medical and Psychological Healers

The initiatory experiences described previously are brief examples of the ways traditional healers in Puerto Rico become both themselves and healers—at the very same time. But we uncovered aspects of this pattern of initiatory experience in the lives of all of the healers in the three groups of women described in this book. However, we also observed that when initiation is condensed into a brief space of time and highly ritualized, it is clearly more intense and impressive, as is the case for most *Espiritistas*. Socialization into biomedical healing also insists upon a confrontation with death through contact with dying patients. It, too, took on impressive meaning as a self-related concern for the young doctors. Similarly, mental health workers who were daily forced to confront bizarre and chaotic behavior in psychotic patients described how they personally experienced the depths of the feeling of nonbeing.

In a way parallel to the *Espiritistas*, other healers reported crisis events, such as the breakup of a marriage or the grave illness of a child or parent, that also pushed them toward the brink of desperation and opened them up to a sense of their own vulnerability. (In my view this course is a central element in initiatory experience.) Yet their development as healers was not identified or given meaning by colleagues. It tended therefore to be perceived as a serendipitous series of life events rather than a transformative process with a purposeful direction. These meaningful events took on value only when we asked the doctors and other health professionals why they chose their careers.

In our discussions, Hector and I referred to Ann Ulanov (1981:15), who speaks about the "receiving woman" as a woman "who can receive herself, receive what is other than herself and also be received by others." Such a woman can reject the traditional feminine role stereotypes of wife and mother and be only what she is. She can also reject newer role patterns, such as activist and career woman. The receiving woman can instead grasp to herself other essential attributes of her personal reality, such as power, aggression, spirituality, and earthiness. These qualities have virtually been formally denied to women in traditional Latin societies. Becoming a healer of any type seems to give these attributes space in which to live—although often they only barely manifest.

We agreed that times are changing for women who have acquired professional status. Two medical doctors were able to say, "Being a woman has not at all interfered with my becoming a doctor." But another reported: "I think that in general male doctors resent women doctors. They don't accept the idea that a woman can be competent, and they would prefer her to stay at home. Male doctors sometimes counsel that she shouldn't go into certain specialties that are only for men." It seemed to us that the day has yet to come when women are encouraged and allowed to receive all of themselves.

Conclusion

We suggest that development as a healer of any type can be viewed as a special process in which a woman learns how to receive. She first learns the need for humility and the value of personal experience, because she has begun to receive her own identity. For Spiritists *guías* represent attributes women must receive to be complete—attributes that they have found difficult to acknowledge or that have eluded them in the course of ordinary life experiences. Receiving a powerful doctor as a cooperating spirit who will assist in diagnosing physical illness and will recommend herbal remedies suggests the incorporation of the doctor's status as well as his knowledge. Receiving an earthy *madama* who can bluntly and blatantly talk about sexual matters (in the face of the heavy taboo on doing so, especially in mixed company) is tantamount to developing a connection with the sexual aspect of one's being. In one healer's definition: "A spiritual guide is a being with a certain clarity, with a certain light, that is, it transmits this light to us, helping the person. Because when we see a person and capture certain things about her, we are not ourselves, but we are a medium through which this spirit manifests." The meaning behind this statement is that the *guías* come as a result of a healer's learning how to wait, how to submit to a larger reality—a sacred reality from which the "light" of understanding and feeling comes and can be received.

A politically radical, feminist friend often harangues about submission to the spiritual. She views it as passivity and avoidance of strong action that could bring about a better world for women. Although I acknowledge that it is true that *guías* are talked about as separate from the medium-healer's physical self, the notion of self-as-spirit includes them. The *guías* are an autobiographical storehouse of self-related, core elements of psyche. They are integral to healer-women's life histories as spiritual conceptions. Most are birthed in pain, but they are almost always received in joy. With their assistance, a woman learns how to receive herself as well as others and thus acquire self-awareness—which may or may not lead to immediate social action. But the sustaining belief of all of the women healers, as they expressed it, is that the heartfelt, daily practice of receiving others' distress represents "a small grain of sand" in filling the oceanic void in humanity's present state of chaos.

Notes

1. Anna was in New York at the time, where Spiritism has been syncretized with *Santería*, a practice referred to as Mesa Blanca, which includes worshipping Afro-Christian saints (see Garrison, 1977a).

2. One might interpret Anna's convulsions as an outlet in a safe place for seething anger; her current life is very difficult because both her daughter and husband are psychiatrically ill.

3. The *guías* seem equivalent to Jung's concept of archetypes (see Koss, 1987).

4. Garrison's interest in suggesting such equivalences is practical; her aim is to foster better understanding of the Spiritist belief system on the part of health and mental health professionals. With respect to Spiritist beliefs approached ethnopsychologically, however, the equivalence of Spiritist notions and a psychoanalytic model of the self seems inaccurate.

4

Healers' Work

How do we deal with pain? By turning toward this wounding, by accepting it and developing a personal feeling toward it, we use it and overcome it rather than let it overcome us.

—Ann Belford Ulanov, *Receiving Woman*

How does healing work? What intervenes to relieve pain in the absence of, or in addition to, physical or chemical manipulation of the inner or outer body? What are the special ways in which healers become the vehicles through which healing occurs? This chapter focuses on what biomedical and traditional healers do and on their perceptions and experiences of helping people in pain.

The healing processes popularly accepted in most of the Western world are based upon one of two principles. They are either allopathic, employing treatments based on remedies that produce effects that are different from those caused by the disease or problem, or homeopathic, treating symptoms by medicines or other techniques that produce effects similar to those caused by the disease or problem. Treatment modalities in modern biomedicine are increasingly allopathic in principle, with some few exceptions in the area of preventive medicine, such as vaccination. Psychiatric treatment has always differed from other medical specialties in that it is based in part on a psychodynamic approach and focuses on the psyche as well as on the body (Groesbeck, 1975). Developed within biomedicine, psychoanalysis first relied on the reliving of emotionally traumatic experiences bit by bit, working toward a more adaptive integration of distressing childhood experiences; but more recently it is concerned with the self and relational themes. Other psychological treatments frequently follow homeopathic principles by employing such techniques as desensitization therapy for phobias and behavior modification for antisocial acting out. In addition, psychology attempts to take all disturbances—physical, emotional, and cognitive—into account in the treatment process.

As illustrated by the descriptions of Spiritist healing in the preceding chapter, Spiritism is based more on homeopathic than on allopathic principles.

It seeks to eliminate pain and upset by bringing to the session *causa* spirits held responsible for distressing the client. These spirits mirror and magnify the sufferer's distress through vivid, symbolic, and emotional descriptions of transgressions in present or past lives. The Spiritist healer's expectation, similar to that of some depth psychologists and psychoanalysts, is that confronting pain with pain leads to its ultimate alleviation. Bringing the *causa* spirit to confront the patient is often a painful process for the healer as well as the client. He or she usually experiences the physical pain and distress of the client in his or her own body, which is referred to as *plasmar* (to mold or form) or *captar* (to capture) the spirit.

Women bring an especially "sharp consciousness of pain to this enterprise" of healing (Ulanov, 1981:151). Habituation to pain is composed of two intertwined strands of feminine experience. One is the common experience of denial of one's talents and worth and sometimes even of self-denial of primary identity, of being a woman. This strand is a response to social conventions that lead to the subordination of women in all but the home sphere, and sometimes there as well. The second strand is made up of the physical and psychological suffering that women are heirs to through their physiology. Their experience of suffering is intimately related to the reproductive system as it cycles through normal life developments, reaching *menarche*, childbirth, and finally menopause. The special cultural patterning of reproductive experience in Puerto Rico and elsewhere seems to connect women to healing roles.

If pain and distress are the primordial materials in which therapy must be anchored, as asserted by some of the great psychological healers of recent times, women may have great capacity to become healers. How and if they relate to this basic aspect of their selves differs according to their early experience as well as prescribed patterns of socialization into the healer role. Not only the medium-healers but also the mental health workers and women physicians described in this book cherish ideals and notions about aspects of healing and suffering that were not taught to them as part of the complex, allopathic paradigm into which they were socialized as trainees.

Doctors' View of Healing Work

Apart from what is considered the "real" work of medicine, which is to change or repair physical and physiological processes in the body to restore health or palliate pain and impairment, young women doctors spontaneously expressed to us the idea that the vehicle for therapeutic change is their relationship with each of their patients. And they readily described what they felt this relationship should be. Above all, the patient "should have trust (*confianza*) in the doctor," and yet "see the doctor as a human being." Most important, this should be a relationship of "respect" (*respeto*), a word in

Puerto Rico that is a potent, emotionally charged descriptor of human relations. "Respect" must go in both directions. By this it is meant that each party to the doctor-patient relationship must look for both understanding and appreciation of the other's point of view as well as of the other's essential identity, that is, who each one is, without social or professional trappings. In the physician's view, "respect" in relation to patients can potentially diminish the inevitable perceptions of social distance that arise between uneducated patients and highly trained doctors.

Ideally, doctors "should be simpler and less sophisticated." The woman who said this went on to say that sometimes she became aggressive when patients told her what she should do. "Although I know only a little, it is more than they know." Although this seems to contradict the notion of equal respect that this doctor had just espoused, it was further explained by the comment of another doctor: "The ideal situation is that patients will be understanding, that they will see the doctor as human and possessing faults." Most of these young women shared this view, which pointed to their discomfort at being thought of as omnipotent. They appeared acutely aware of their personal limitations as medical "healers." Although doctors acknowledged that they must rely upon their extensive knowledge and on adequate communication to help patients, at the same time they were uncertain about what qualities of the doctor-patient relationship could enhance their healing task and how they might use such qualities.

We thought that some of the doctors' confusion could be due to their neophyte status. What was somewhat curious (but may not be, given their participation in our project) were their favorable views on Spiritism. They all wanted to understand more about it, and almost all agreed that patients who "believed" could be helped by an *Espiritista*, if the illness was "psychosomatic" or "emotional." Awilda said, "If one is unable to arrive at a diagnosis for someone's symptoms, then perhaps a doctor can refer that patient to an *Espiritista*." Another doctor said, "Patients see medicine as an alternative for their health problems," but "sometimes they resort to traditional medicine in desperation." Anna felt that "perhaps *Espiritistas* do not have (medical) knowledge, but they do have the will to help."

Although it is possible that their openness to Spiritism indicates doubt about the efficacy of biomedicine among young physicians, it could also relate to the family backgrounds of these particular women, all of whom had had some contact with Spiritist healing through mothers or other close female relatives. Several had resorted to Spiritists themselves when faced with personal crises in recent years. One woman was open about her belief in Spiritism and had had personal confirmation of spirit phenomena. Two others shared some Spiritist beliefs and were willing to say that "spirits exist" and "reincarnation is a fact." Although this group is self-selected in terms of interest in Spiritism, interviews with a number of physicians in Puerto Rico frequently produced the same openness, particularly if their mothers or other relatives believed in or practiced Spiritism. As described in more detail elsewhere (Koss, 1980), a small number of doctors in Puerto Rico are also Spiritist healers. They either incorporate a few Spiritist techniques into their allopathic medical practices or regularly attend *centros* in the role of Spiritist healers, completely apart from their medical practices. One doctor in the Project reported that she knew that "the development of Spiritism in Latin America had paralleled that of Western medicine during the nineteenth century." For her, this fact made it possible to consider Spiritism a viable alternative, even for the scientifically trained professional.

I do not think that the involvement of these doctors in Spiritism is merely the result of geographic or familial access to its practices. Despite medical training as rigorous as that found in the United States, world- and self-views expressed by Puerto Ricans include Spiritist notions as culturally rationalized beliefs, proven by experience. Thus, to act upon Spiritist beliefs in one's private life is a conflict-free choice for some medical professionals, especially when these beliefs proceed out of early family relationships.

Mental Health Workers' View of Their Healing Work

Women mental health professionals came from a variety of disciplines, having been trained as nurses, social workers, psychologists, or in nonclinical disciplines in the behavioral sciences. They were rather eclectic in the ways they viewed and treated their patients but agreed upon an almost missionary-like attitude toward the relief of suffering. This view, primarily allopathic in perspective, was suffused with the need to stop pain and distress rapidly. However, their common use of counseling therapies more often belied than realized the ideal allopathic perspective. This approach was in fact encouraged by the explicit policies of the community mental health division of the Puerto Rican Health Department, which de-emphasized the use of psychotropic drugs, especially tranquilizers, in favor of individual or group therapy, day care, or partial hospitalization for clients diagnosed as chronically mentally ill.

To illustrate how mental health professionals worked with their clients, I present brief summaries of two typical cases, focusing on therapists' descriptions of how they dealt with a particular patient and on the generalizations they made about how they usually worked.

Milagros, a social worker, prefaced her description of her work with a sixty-year-old male client, whom she had seen over a number of months, with the following remarks:

> As a social worker, always when I see a person sitting in front of me who is seeking help, I take a moment to remember that I am in front of a human being who has had a lot of experiences, some convictions, some anxieties. My first obligation is to try to see what is the situation of the client, patient, or person in order to try to gauge the nature of the relationship [with me]; what is going to be my technique to help him, with what I have to deal in order to understand him, to be able to enter into his world and help him to deal with his difficulties as much as possible.

This attitude was quite common among the mental health workers, reflecting notions similar to those of the medical doctors, particularly with regard to the ideal that the therapist must "respect" the patient. Our observations confirmed that this ideal was honored by most mental health workers whenever allowed by the institutional arrangements under which they worked. However, frustrations frequently broke through and the ideal was forgotten when a patient seemed uncooperative or noncompliant. Because most mental health professionals carried very large caseloads, from one hundred and fifty to two hundred patients, they generally saw a client only once a month. We observed that the insufficiency of time in relation to most patients' needs often left the therapists unable to observe progressive changes. Hence frustration was common.

According to Milagros:

> Don Juan had been married for thirty-two years and had six children between the ages of twenty-two and thirty years. He had only married once, was Catholic, and had finished the sixth year of elementary school. He was a worker in pineapples and sugar cane; later a vendor in a small business, was in the army for two years, but didn't leave Puerto Rico. His last job was working as a mechanic for farm equipment. Two years and two months previously he had returned from work, claiming nervousness. He attributed his illness to work conditions, retired for incapacity, and was referred to the Social Security office (*Fondo del Seguro del Estado*).
>
> He presented the following symptoms:
>
> He felt very nervous (*mal de los nervios*), he couldn't sleep, he didn't want to leave the house, preferred to be alone. He also had a problem with his youngest son, who had been apprehended for selling marijuana three times. He felt desperate. His goal in coming to find help was "to feel better and be tranquil." Other physical symptoms presented were pain in his chest, and he said he suffered from high blood pressure. He had strong, frequent headaches and also suffered from varicose veins.

Milagros described to the assembled group how Don Juan had sought help at various hospitals and was referred to the mental health center when the Veterans' Hospital ruled that his nervous condition was not service connected. She went on to describe how Don Juan felt nervous for three or four months before he left his job, but also how she came to "use this situation [his illness] to stimulate him to analyze all of the circumstances surrounding it, to look at all of the positive things in his life, and to clarify other possible causes of his nervousness." Through this indirect method, that is, encouraging him to talk openly about his problems (because she felt he was not accustomed to doing so at home), she identified the central problem that was bothering him. Although his son had not been incarcerated and had returned to school, this man was deeply worried over a fee payment to the lawyer who had defended the boy. Two of his daughters managed to support the household in which he lived, and he had some income from his small farm, but there was not enough to pay the debt to the lawyer. Milagros then seized upon this last problem, specifically Don Juan's discomfort over making a commitment "under false premises" (in Don Juan's words), because he thought he was going to receive a veteran's disability pension. Milagros then worked out a way for the family to repay the debt. She noted (in her words, "she captured") that the relationship between her and her client was strengthened; it seemed likely that Don Juan would "now bring out other things he had at the back of his mind" because he now had confidence in her. Milagros stressed how she usually worked to bring about growth of trust (*confianza*) when it sometimes took "as long as fourteen sessions." She commented: "For me . . . it is very important to cultivate a positive feeling (*sembrar una semilla positiva*). In doing that I am working less materialistically and I am seeing into his spiritual side . . . into his values, into his emotions, so that he will live a happy life."

She then clarified the treatment plan for this client. She was waiting to see what else would arise in therapy, and she planned to eliminate further difficulties as they arose.

After the session in which Milagros presented her case, Hector and I discussed how the allopathic paradigm of elimination of pain to assist the client to a state of happy equilibrium was aptly illustrated in her case discussion. She had given voice to the basic assumption that this man's dignity was her point of departure. She then permitted his conception of his problems to come into the sessions. She also reported that she "treated the environment," that is, she brought familial relationships into their work as a way to help Don Juan "count his blessings." She said further that this was accomplished through the "awareness that he had his basic needs taken care of, that is, his clothing, food, and medical care, and he had a family that loved him."

We felt that Milagros's approach reflected both her training as a social worker and her own personal style. She was a middle-aged woman and had a distinctly maternal way of dealing with her clients. As noted earlier, carrying out the mother role as a therapist is an easy, "natural" path for most Puerto Rican women, especially when they are over forty years of age. We often observed that the special veneer of professionalism that seems common in the United States is just beginning to be acquired by some Puerto Rican women.

At another case review session, the presenter was Nelda, a twenty-nine-year-old woman who had trained as a psychologist at the University of Puerto Rico and had earned her master's degree four years prior to our study. In her approach to her patients, as she described it, Nelda appeared more systematic and formal than did Milagros. At that session Nelda presented the case of Diana.

> Forty-three years old, single, Catholic and a secretary, she was referred by a friend. Her principal complaint was a "current" on her left side starting from her head. When she touched that side it hurt and continued to do so even when she didn't touch it. The doctors couldn't find anything. [Nelda then detailed the number of laboratory tests Diana had had, none of which turned up evidence of a physical problem.] The patient related that she had lived in the U.S., in New York, for eleven years. She went to New York because her father abandoned her mother and she had to take responsibility for the family. She found good employment as an interpreter for a social worker and worked there for a long time, functioning very well. Before this time, her life in Puerto Rico had been more or less quiet. She didn't have any of these symptoms. After about seven years, she decided to come to Puerto Rico for vacation and stayed with a relative. Diana recalled that she had had a nightmare that an iguana was attached to her left shoulder with tape. And some persons in the dream said, "No one is going to help you take this off." And in the dream she said, "Yes, I will find someone." And she began to walk in her dream and ask for help in all of the houses, but no one would help her, and people laughed.
>
> Diana then returned to the U.S. One day, while taking a cake out of the oven, she suffered an "attack" (*ataque de nervios*). She then left her job, returned to Puerto Rico, and found work for five years but continued to suffer the "shooting" pain in her left side. She had to stop working because of the pain.

Nelda went on to describe Diana's family history. Her parents had divorced over a disagreement about her father's becoming a Pentecostal church member; the family had refused to accept the father's new rules. However, Diana was later left burdened with the responsibility for her mother and younger siblings, including a blind brother.

Nelda then detailed her interventions with Diana, beginning with helping her list the problems on which she wanted to work. Nelda's next step was to formulate a hypothesis about the cause of her client's problems. Besides "depression and anxiety," Nelda assessed Diana's problems to be "existential," that is, she "was suffering from a midlife crisis and badly regretted her lost life."

Nelda uncovered the story of a lover who had left Diana to marry another woman. Diana met this man again at the time of the iguana dream, which she felt was a prediction of her current pain. He told her he regretted having married someone else, but he could do nothing about it. When Nelda confronted Diana with this information as a possible source of her distress, Diana did not accept the theory that it had caused her problem. Nelda felt that Diana was "denying," that is, using "unconscious defenses" to deal with her problems. But on checking her hypothesis, she found that Diana currently had a boyfriend (*novio*) and was planning to marry. On consideration, Nelda felt that Diana had developed "a pattern of unconscious defenses" against seeing the reality of her life situation, which would be "difficult to break" because it had gone on for over five years. But Nelda said she felt the prognosis to be favorable. Diana could be "cured" because she had shown she was aware of the nature of her problems and could accept them. Moreover, she could manage life adequately and function well. Nelda placed a high value on Diana's capacity to take on responsibilities and to find a male partner. We interpreted this to mean that Diana had demonstrated that she could successfully manage what Nelda believed were a woman's most important life tasks.

Two other facets of Nelda's treatment plan were interesting for the light they shed on her view of how she worked with patients and on how she thought about therapeutic success. Using a psychiatric diagnostic manual (DSMII, American Psychiatric Association, 1968; this was the policy of the Community Mental Health Center where Nelda worked), Nelda labeled Diana's condition as "reactive depression with features of anxiety." Nelda said she thought that Diana's anxiety was related to the "existential" question "What have I done with my life?" Nelda told her audience that the label "reactive" indicated a condition of relatively short duration associated with specific precipitating events. Once the problems associated with these events were solved, the condition could be "cured."

A second important aspect of Nelda's formulation and review of this case was her description of her relationship with Diana as close to "ideal." "She is a person who is very cooperative in the therapy, and she is much desirous of understanding herself, of becoming aware of some things for herself." Nelda described how she used certain techniques with Diana that she could not use with other patients who were less "sophisticated." She praised Diana because she felt that Diana didn't force her to provide medications. Because of these "favorable" aspects of the therapeutic relationship, particularly Diana's active participation in her therapy, Nelda said that she was able to use

Gestalt therapy (Perls, 1951). This, she explained, was a way to relate all of the Diana's subpersonalities to various actions and events.

Just "talking with her patients" was therapeutic, according to Nelda's presentation. She described how her clients got better because they were forced to deal with things that they had never dealt with before; they were "learning to see themselves a little bit more and to know themselves a little bit better." Moreover, "it helps lessen tensions, and [the patient] can share things she has never been able to share with other persons."

We knew from interviewing her that Nelda was very familiar with the limitations of the community mental health system in Puerto Rico and acknowledged that she was able to treat many of her patients in a "more sophisticated" way because she had the luxury of having only a few. We observed that those therapists with large caseloads had to be more efficient, and therefore they worked at a level that Nelda described (and we observed) as very "realistic." Their approach to a patient was often, "This is your problem, what are you going to do about it?" And, "How will you do it?" They worked much more in crisis-oriented ways with acutely disturbed clients and also offered support for clients suffering chronic mental illness. Everyone in the CMHCs mentioned at one time or another that long-term psychotherapy was not feasible.

The Work of Spiritists

In our discussions of healing in Spiritism we observed that one must consider the phenomenon of sufferers being "healed" by becoming healers themselves as distinct from the ways in which Spiritists deal with persons they do not diagnose as "in development." Some *centros* hold special weekly sessions to assist mediums-in-development. Whereas "development" is considered a lifelong condition—more difficult at its inception than later—other types of spirit-caused distress (such as difficulty with a spirit coming from a past incarnation, problems with one's own spirit, or being *encadenada* [tied to a chain of disturbed spirits and unable to break free of this entanglement]), usually require only short-term attention and are generally worked on in one or perhaps a few sessions.

We were fascinated by the observation that once having developed faculties, the knowledge (and feelings) acquired from this experience acts as an inner teacher of the healing process itself. A number of therapeutic modalities employ this principle, from Alcoholics Anonymous to the psychoanalytic psychologies. Moreover, as we had observed and read, when an ill person is treated by a group, the environment becomes an integral part of the therapeutic process by providing an arena of social support in which being "well" is associated with control over illness or distress. Both the ill state and the process of transcending it (that is, of being "healed") take on social meaning.

People thus healed then assume the special role and status of healers. In Alcoholics Anonymous, for example, the "recovering alcoholic" becomes the teacher and mentor of those still unrecovered or "immoral" because they are alcoholic.

We observed that the same pattern obtains for *Espiritistas*. Once symptoms of an illness become known to relatives or close friends who believe in Spiritism, whether or not the symptoms are recognized at first as "development," the ill person may be taken to a *centro*. If diagnosed as "in development of faculties," an informal apprenticeship takes place in which the novitiate is told to sit at the table beside the practicing medium-healers and report her experiences as part of the healing session. She is also assigned rituals to carry out at home, consisting of prayers, readings from Kardec's books or other Spiritist writings, and meditation exercises. These practices focus on finding out more about one's spirit *cuadro* (repertoire) of guides.

Recalling this time in her life, Mili spoke of how "Spiritism came upon me without my wanting it to and without my knowing what it was. I became anxious if I didn't go to the temples. I preferred the temples to parties. I became too scared to have *videncias* [evidence of spirits, usually images], so I didn't. [Instead] I saw things in my mind. I have many dreams and I work in the dreams. I see many beautiful places and am transported to places where needed."

Mili said that the first time she had an experience of spirits coming through her, she was at her mother-in-law's house. She felt something strange and began to scream. "I felt compelled to speak out, but it [the spirit] wouldn't let me. A girl came in whose mother had died when she was born. (I saw her later in a dream.) I talked a lot when this happened and moved my hands. My heart started to beat rapidly, and when I felt my chest was going to open out, then I began to speak because that gave me strength to speak. I spoke then until that [feeling] stopped."

Sara, the research assistant on the Project, experienced trance for the first time and reported:

> I was motionless, and moving became entirely difficult. I was unable to concentrate, and this was made worse by the fact that I was frightened. I started to get as if it were a headache. Then I felt a rush of warmth throughout my body. I seemed to be losing awareness of my surroundings, as if becoming ambivalent and my senses weakened. All of a sudden I felt like something inside me, sort of disassociated with myself, wanted to make me pound my fist on the table and start talking.

Sara was at a session at the time and reported to us that she told the head medium about her distress while frantically trying not to lose consciousness. Doña Josephina dipped her hands into the bowl of "fluidized" water on the table and held them in front of Sara's face while moving them in a circular motion. In her field notes Sara wrote:

> I watched her hands intently with my eyes, following their movement. Then she took my hands in hers and moved my arms while making me stand up with her. This movement was also circular. Then she flung my arms out and I started falling backwards because of the strength of her flinging motion, or because I was coming out of that trance. She then took the spirit as it were, and it turned out that the spirit wanted to interrupt what the other spirit was talking about.

We discussed how, in both of these cases, the feelings of going "under" and losing control, of having to rely upon another person who was wiser and stronger in dealing with the unknown, while at the same time acknowledging one's vulnerability to mysterious forces within one's own consciousness, all appeared to become significant parts of the development of the self in those who underwent development of faculties. Mili's taking on the spirit of a woman who had died in childbirth, whose identity as a nurse she later discovered in a dream, illustrates the type of symbolic image that can speak to the birth of a woman's identity.

Mili recalled that her first experience with trance had occurred at a time when she was struggling to overcome personal and social obstacles in order to acquire professional training. She had planned to study nursing but married at nineteen years of age and then had to work in factories for a number of years. The experience of falling into a trance state at a *centro* brought her into closer relationships with her mother and mother-in-law, both of whom believed in Spiritism and practiced it regularly. Most important, these trance experiences meant that she had to depend upon an older woman healer to guide her through the chaos of development. We observed that sometimes this dependence is diffused among a group of mediums at a particular *centro*, but most often one woman, usually the "president of the table" who has organized the group, assumes the role of spiritual mentor for all those in development in her *centro*. After reviewing the life histories of many women just before one project seminar, we discussed how this connection with a "healer-mother" seems to take up the mothering task where one's own mother has left off. This seems to be true particularly when a mother has not been able to model the strength and self-esteem needed to achieve those accomplishments that bring a woman a sense of empowerment.

Therapeutic Relationships

In our discussions we noted that therapeutic relationships are born out of a number of choices that any healer (of any type) must make with regard to a patient or client. A healer can remain aloof and phrase all of her interventions in a nonpersonal, indirect way. This was illustrated by Nelda's comment about the necessity for efficiency and the time constraints that are common for many mental health workers. These constraints prompt them to confront their clients knowing that their responsibility is to take immediate action to relieve their clients' problems. Or healers can be very directive in handing down advice or prescriptions without ever entering into the feelings and perceptions of the client. This was the paradox first pointed out by the medical doctors who participated in the Project. Ideally, these doctors could possess all of the knowledge necessary to help a patient, but they were afraid that patients would expect too much, even miracles, that they could never produce. The women physicians often said that they longed to have a relationship of "mutual respect" with their patients but also recognized that they needed *confianza* (trust) from their patients in order to effectively exercise their healing skills.

We speculated that perhaps because of the extensive training and knowledge required for the practice of medical and psychological healing, there is all too frequently a tendency for health professionals to derogate patients or clients who arrive in such severe distress that they exhibit regressive behavior and heightened dependency needs. Yet we observed that patients or clients in their turn may be quite ready to submit to being directed by someone who can offer hope of relief from the threat of illness or personal dissolution. It seems that patients are viewed even more negatively if differences in social class and prestige are perceived by the physicians or mental health professionals. Even though the ideology of social equality is widely espoused in Puerto Rico, class differences based on education, money, and skin color are important guidelines in social interactions (Safa, 1975). The perception of social class difference mutually affects patients and health professionals, varying somewhat with how the health professionals identify their own social statuses.

Spiritist Healer-Client Relationships

We often observed that the advent of an initiatory illness in a client, as well as a first experience of alteration of consciousness in the ritual setting, poses the difficult problem of often extreme dependence upon a particular Spiritist healer.[1] The psychoanalytic model of transference provides an interesting parallel. In psychoanalysis the patient's life becomes entwined with a projected image of the analyst. Working through earlier traumas or complexes inhibiting a comfortable life adaptation in part depends upon the "working out" of the dependence upon the analyst, who is a nurturing paternal or maternal figure. What is called "individuation" in analysis is based upon breaking the dependency that therapy engenders in terms of much-longed-for experiences of acceptance and belonging.

Healing "work" among Spiritist healers depends upon reciprocal relationships with their guide-protector spirits. We observed that, quite apart from their significance as newly discovered, newly integrated, part-selves, the *guías* are extremely important for developing healers, who have dependency needs and who come to rely more and more upon the *guías*. The presence of the *guías* as powerful allies in the new medium-healers' consciousness of self is the way Spiritism resolves the basic paradox of therapies whose purpose is personal transformation. These therapies heighten dependency but insist upon the development of an autonomous sense of self. The *guías* were described by the medium-healers as assisting their clients "in development" to become aware of personal power for decision making and action in the world.

We were told, however, that *guías* do not automatically permit a relationship of dependence and submission in exchange for their supportive help in healing internal malaise or interpersonal conflict. *Guías* exact a price for both their intimacy and assistance. They insist that the healer not offend them by behaving in ways they disapprove and ultimately that she (or he) recognize her own negative characteristics and faults. Most important, they demand that Spiritist mediums eternally continue their spirit work. We were often told by Spiritist healers that to stop working at the table risks the probability of relapsing into a state of illness. Several women in this group of healers attempted other religious healing practices at times during their lives, such as becoming active in the Pentecostal Church. But these women told us that they eventually were forced to return to Spiritism and to their healing work because they had fallen seriously ill.

Almost every healer explained that once having received her *guías* they taught her a number of specific skills. Most mediums are *videntes*; they said, that is, mediums can see "with an inner eye" what is occurring in the spirit world on behalf of a client. This is only one source of knowledge about the spirit world, a "clear-sightedness" that provides "evidence" of the evolutionary track of each spirit. Other sources of knowledge (called *facultades*) include hearing spirits; seeing them in dreams or through "intuition," "clairvoyance," or knowing what will happen in the future; *desdoble*, being able to project one's spirit-consciousness to another place when needed; and *plasmar*, capturing another's pain or feelings in one's own body. Some mediums described how they feel the fluids around the patient in order to work with the "subtle" or "etheric" body.

We observed that healers sometimes prescribed baths of herbs and perfumed oils or herbal teas. In individual sessions, as well as *centros*, they also counseled clients around practical matters, such as marital conflict or a court case. And, most demanding of all, they regularly received spirits into their bodies (which they referred to as "material envelopes"), thus permitting the spirits to speak through them. This last skill was referred to as "passing" the *causa* spirits, who are "ignorant," "confused," "bad," "backward," and inevitably attracted to the spirit *cuadros* of those persons who have not yet evolved. As described earlier, the *causas* are difficult to "receive," especially when they possess and speak through the medium-healers. Many healers say they do not develop as *mediunidades parlantes* (speaking mediums) because they are afraid to take the *causa* spirits into their bodies because these spirits "cut" them.

Hector and I often discussed how the faculty of *plasmando* or *captando* (molding or capturing) what another person is feeling is of special interest for understanding the difference between Spiritist healing practices and medical and psychological healing. The quality and nature of the ritual encounter between a Spiritist healer and her client are reflected in the extent to which they mutually enter into the client's experience of illness or distress. (See, for example, LeShan, 1974.) We felt that one could say that the Spiritist healer identifies completely with the client's spiritual condition and endeavors to create or to open a therapeutic space where they meet as one. Thus "faculties," as experienced by the medium, contribute to bringing about a sense of identification between client and healer. For example, by the medium's "taking" into her body the *causa* spirit affecting her client or through feelings aroused when the spiritual "fluids" pass between her and her client, a channel for intimacy and closeness is opened between them. At most sessions, we observed that a healer's *guía* will instruct her to tell the client what she or he is feeling. At the very same time, the medium feels these same symptoms within her own body. Her experience of the client's symptoms is then expressed in a physical idiom, such as "you have a pain in your lower back" or "you feel a heaviness in the bronchial tubes." More rarely it is expressed in a kind of psychological idiom, such as "your mind is blank," "you want to abandon your family," or "you feel inferior."

In our musings about how Spiritist healing works, we agreed that the extent of the medium's identification with his or her client's inner experience can be appreciated when the *causa* spirit responsible for causing the client's distress is taken into the healer's body. At the sessions, we had many times seen the gestures accompanied by sounds, grimaces and groans, the shouting, panting, writhing, and limping, the wheezing, clutching, falling backward, and other body-endangering actions with which the healer nonverbally mirrored her client's distress. It was as if the healer were saying: "This is your pain. I too can feel its destructive chaos as its foreign body fills me, but I have developed the strength and knowledge to overcome it."

Of course we had also observed the *causa* spirit speaking through the mouth of the medium-healer and explaining why it was causing the client's pain and discomfort. In our opinion, this gives the sufferer a chance to confront the cause of her distress, mostly through her tangible connection to the spiritual events behind it, but always by the ritual of saying "Te *perdone*" (I forgive you) to the *causa* spirit, which must occur before it will leave the possessed medium-healer. The affective charge of seeing an outer display of one's own inner feelings appears to provide some possibility of detachment from them. The Spiritists said they intend that the suffering client acquire distance from the mire of distress within which she has been caught. (We also observed that this is not always the outcome of the healing encounter.) But we reasoned that the Spiritist healing ritual directs the sufferer to look upon her illness as an inevitable part of a fated life plan for which she must assume some moral responsibility, even though she is not directly responsible for bringing it about.

As the *Espiritistas* told the seminar participants, healer and client equally share in an effort directed by the healer to contact the healing power within themselves. They said that the source of this healing force is called the Holy Spirit, God. Their efforts to *plasmar* the feelings of their clients are said to be arduous, but because the healer has a built-in bodily knowledge of suffering (gained through the initiatory and other illnesses), the process ideally brings relief for both healer and client. As will be described in the following chapter, the healer's opening her body to *causa* spirits is feared as ultimately dangerous to her health and well-being. Ideally, however, her *guías* are there to protect her. They will also make sure that her own spirit can reenter her body, thus assuring her continuity of identity. We interpreted this to mean that it is these newly acquired part-selves, the *guías*, who are responsible for the continuity of the healer's self. They are her most powerful attributes.

The Inner Healer

We had read about "endogenous healing mechanisms" (Prince, 1976), which can account for the effects of nonmedical healing practices but are also constellated in therapeutic relationships (Groesbeck, 1975). There is an extensive literature on the placebo effect (Moerman, 1983) in which a pharmacologically inert substance, after being given to a patient as if it were the appropriate medication, was effective. And there are reports of the alleviation of symptoms, and even of the prolongation of life, following the use of psychological techniques (Pelletier, 1977). These writings all suggest that we possess a kind of "inner healer" (or mechanism) who can help resolve physical ailments and discomfort. The recently discovered endogenous opiates are now known to inhibit pain from within the brain itself (Prince, 1982).

We opined that ritual healing techniques in Spiritism can be viewed physiologically as ways to mobilize endogenous processes within the central nervous systems of clients. They may also be viewed from an experiential perspective as a special variant of the therapeutic relationship, a ritual encounter through which a distressed person in a highly suggestible state can feel a sense of instant intimacy with another being through the sharing of pain and distress. The healer, through action and appearance, is perceived (also apperceived) as manifesting great love and concern. This perspective on the Spiritist healing encounter agrees with that of the *Espiritistas* themselves. They rarely emphasized the "material" causes of the illnesses they saw, although they did employ remedies aimed at physically manipulating the body. For example, María reported that during a session she "captured" the pains of a client who had fallen on her head (in another existence). Later, at her home, she "gave her [client] back and neck massages [*sobos*]" and felt that she had healed her "bones." María later explained that the power of the Holy Spirit came through her as she performed the massages.

In a similar vein, Milagros told the seminar that she had seen a woman who had "fever, diarrhea, was vomiting and unable to eat, and had lost a great deal of weight." This woman had gone to a physician and later to the medical center, but all tests were negative. Her doctor gave up on her and suggested (in exasperation, according to the patient) that she see an *Espiritista.* Milagros told this woman to use herbal baths and teas of the plant molinillo (*Hura crepitans*) for the fever. But the prescription was not based upon the symptoms. The cause of this woman's illness was "seen" to be a cancer from a friend that had "stuck to her" (*se le pego a ella*) when this friend died. The friend's spirit was "looking for help" (*buscando una ayuda*) and had stuck to Milagros's client because she had not been able to visit her before she died. The spirit of the dead friend stayed around because of the client's anxiety over not seeing her friend before she died, but the spirit was not aware that it was harming anyone.

We remarked to the seminar participants that in this case the herbal preparations were like placebos, but they were not placebos per se because they were not aimed at causing physiological change in the body of the client. Instead they were aimed at helping rid this woman of the illness-causing spirit of her dead friend. Treating the fever was also a means of dealing with the molesting spirit.

Spiritists' and Therapists' Work Compared

The following discussion briefly summarizes a whole series of observations we made as we presided over the Project seminars during September and October 1977. We discussed the fact that the mental health professionals and the *Espiritistas* share a number of approaches to healing, although their different belief systems pose very different models of the world (Garrison, 1979; Koss, 1980). Both psychotherapy and Spiritist healing aim to reduce anxiety; encourage catharsis by permitting patients to acknowledge socially unacceptable emotions; permit dependency and other regressive types of behavior; deal with expressed and nonverbalized guilt feelings by variously blaming problems on parents, social forces, or spirits; encourage the confession of feelings that have been hidden from the sufferer herself; and assist (often, even direct) the search for personal values and meaning.

Mental health workers bring to their professional healing a repertoire of technical models for behavior, but most seem to use them rather eclectically. A few therapists use family therapy, and all work with and counsel family members in relation to a relative's illness. Some have learned techniques of behavior modification and employ these, although not always systematically. Of the various psychological approaches, behavior modification is used most frequently. It is described as appealing to the "concreteness" of thought of most mental health clients who are not "sophisticated." One psychiatrist commented that psychodynamic psychotherapy is not used because of the "tremendous investment of time and money, when the person who comes for help really only wants to rapidly get over the problem." The director of an outpatient clinic, a psychologist, described her approach to treating clients as follows:

> The client says, My problem is with my wife or my son, my daughter. Well, then, she [the mental health worker] is going to deal with this problem specifically. She will solve that problem. . . . We don't enter into considerations of "What are your dreams, what happened when you were small?" If that has some significance in terms of the problem, OK, it is utilized. [But] it is an approach that is more directive. The therapist is less passive and more active. Do you see that?

There is a point beyond which similarities in the approaches of mental health workers and *Espiritistas* seem to disappear. The edge of this difference was described earlier in relation to the way healers and clients relate to each other. The psychotherapeutic relationship was described by Project participants as more "objective," each party maintaining some emotional distance. The specific techniques of psychotherapy are individually adapted tools based on objectively construed models for behavior. They are, however, laced with socially construed notions and prejudices, such as beliefs that clients are "unsophisticated" or "concrete thinkers." This was also seen in mental health workers' expressed views of clients as desiring quick resolution of specific problems rather than wanting to work toward self-knowledge and personal transformation. We concluded that these views were in part responses to the constraints dictated by the community mental health system within which they worked. However, psychologists in private practice in Puerto Rico, who gave lectures at our seminars, also voiced some of the same notions about their patients.

In contrast, although it was common for Spiritists to have only one or two sessions with persons in acute distress, many were prepared to help their clients over long periods of time if needed. They expected long-term personal transformations in persons identified as "in development." "Personal transformation" is our term for what they referred to as "spiritual evolution," a basic Spiritist notion of the human condition. Thus most Spiritists differed from mental health professionals in their willingness to give themselves to their clients and to receive the clients' pain as if it were their own. This difference is illustrated in Nelda's comments about the client who dreamed of the iguana.

> I felt that she was asking a great deal during the therapy. In addition, sometimes I had to invest more time with her than I had planned because in one way she was asking for it. [I thought] well, it's probably because she does not have substitutes in the community. And the last time I saw her I asked, and she explained that she had one friend who did not live in her town, and she had another—that is, her friends were not very accessible.

When we compared this statement with María's account of her work with the mentally ill young woman, we felt that there was a real difference. After two and a half years of seeing her client on a routine basis, María took a two-week vacation. Just after she returned she recalled that

> I encountered the girl's mother in the grocery store and I asked about her girl. The mother, crying, grabbed my arms and told me. "Ay, María, she is always crying; she wants to see you; she wants to return to you." Then, thanks to God, who gave me this spirit and willpower that I have always had for this [work]; and also my spiritual strengths, well, I said, "Look, I am willing to deal with her. See if the hospital will release her or give her a pass." I told them that I would work with the girl. That was Friday. The mother went and already by Saturday the girl was on leave from the hospital, happy that she was going to see me.

We also observed that there was an important difference between the Spiritists and the therapists in their ideas about sources of knowledge on how to heal. The therapists constantly spoke about a book or a theory or a system of doing therapy as providing them with guidelines for working with patients. They were uncomfortable when the *Espiritistas* supported their therapeutic judgments with "evidence" they saw in the world of the spirits. In practice, however, both groups of healers mostly worked out of their personally rich experiential storehouses (with the exception, perhaps, of the medical doctors). These differences were obvious only when the healers were called upon to explain what they did.

We identified and labeled two different attitudes—the scientific/objective and the experiential/subjective—because they did seem to make an important difference in relationships with patients and clients. The *Espiritistas* did not expect a client to describe her problems before the *Espiritista* received a "picture" or feelings about the client's pain or distress and could then check out this evidence with the client. The major approach of the *Espiritistas* was to "open" the spiritual space of clients who came to their sessions or consultations through meditative prayer and the creation of a sense of general comfort and well-being. They concerned themselves with receiving their clients in particular ways: with coffee and warmth when in their homes; with peace, love, and concern when in their *centros*. Thus, in essence, they personally and ritually set the stage for healing events to occur rather than act upon a patient or situation. In this sense, much more was expected of Spiritist healers with regard to taking the initial responsibility for knowing about patients and investing in their bodies, spirits, and emotions.

In contrast, we observed that mental health workers felt forced to take an active role with patients, who, in turn, were expected to disclose their pain, distress, and confidences before they could be helped. This "objective" attitude (as the mental health workers labeled it) appeared to convey the message that medical doctors and mental health workers should be immune to the distress of their patients. They told us how their trainers and role models encouraged them to develop defenses against emotional involvement, and they more or less did so. In actual practice, however, many health professionals (as illustrated by the young doctors' comments at the beginning of this chapter) often personally assumed the responsibility for curing even terminally ill patients, which contrasted with the Spiritists, who were sure that God was ultimately responsible for patients they could not help.

Although the preceding discussion might give the impression that we favor the Spiritists as more effective in helping to cope with emotional distress, it is clear to us that effectivity is a complex issue and its measurement subject to many variations in construct and content, according to the talent and skill of the individual healer. Elsewhere I present data on the self-reported effectiveness of Spiritists as compared with therapists (Koss, 1987). I show that Spiritists are reported to be more successful in relieving some complaints, but therapists are more effective with other complaints, while they both do equally well with the majority of complaints women present. In summary, it can be said that all types of healers seemed to experience the same joy when successful, and all suffered some personal distress when their healing work failed. The doctors and the mental health workers in the Project appeared to us to be somewhat better defended by the professional codes and ethics that governed their relationships with patients and by their veil of objectivity, although at times this was more an ideal than a reality. The only defense the Spiritists used was to conduct most of their healing work in groups—and this, too, had its negative side, as will be seen in the next chapter. The already "wounded" Spiritist healers expressed and reported more vulnerability to illness and distress than the health professionals—a vulnerability that we felt was inherent in the choice of vocation or avocation as a healer.

Notes

1. I have written in detail about the problem of dependence and its transcendence in an early article. See Koss, 1975.

5

The Distaff Side: Pitfalls and Problems of Being a Healer

Among laymen one frequently meets with the prejudice that psychotherapy is the easiest thing in the world and consists in the art of putting something over on people or wheedling money out of them. But actually it is a tricky and not undangerous calling. Just as doctors are exposed to infections and other occupational hazards, so the psychotherapist runs the risk of psychic infections which are no less menacing. On the one hand he is often in danger of getting entangled in the neuroses of his patients; on the other hand if he tries too hard to guard against their influence, he robs himself of his therapeutic efficacy. Between this Scylla and this Charybdis lies the peril, but also the healing power.

—C. G. Jung, *Collected Works*

None of the healers in our Project ever spoke with regret about becoming a healer or voiced the desire to change her choice of vocation or avocation. Their satisfaction was expressed in a number of ways: in particular, they all appeared avidly interested in their patients, clients, and work and seemed to enjoy the opportunity to discuss their experiences. As noted earlier, all said they found personal meaning in helping others, and a few doctors and mental health workers mentioned other kinds of rewards, such as higher social status and salary. The Spiritist healers expressed an even more intense attitude in that they said they felt compelled to their healing task by implicit threats to maintaining their own health and well-being. But all of the healers, when participating in or discussing healing practices in the seminars or during our interviews, gave the impression that they experienced intermittent but intense satisfaction and sometimes even joy and ecstasy. Despite these positive rewards, there were difficulties in being a woman and healer, which were different for each of the healer groups and most serious for Spiritists, whose lives did not merely contain their healing roles but were instead contained by them.

From discussions with the healers we found that the routes to these difficulties, though intertwined, originated in several sources. The most important was the social valuation of femininity in Puerto Rico. One can best describe how women are perceived by using the psychological concept of "ambivalence." Much has been written about Latin male attitudes toward women (often referred to in the social science literature as part of the *machismo* image). Men's notions about women generally dichotomize into idealizing them as virtuous, passive, virginal beings, and vilifying them as immoral, lascivious whores (Acosta-Belen, 1980). Although Puerto Rican men say they desire and do obtain virgin brides, many, if not most, seem to be avidly and continually searching for (or serving) experienced, sexually active lovers (*queridas*). Although seldom openly discussed, the phenomenon of the "mistress," an often not-so-secret woman on the side, is common and not altogether unexpected by older and middle-aged wives. (It is now much less tolerated by younger, working women.)

We often commented on the fact that although the developing economy is allowing greater numbers of women to join the work force, this has not changed the pattern of marital relations to any extent, except perhaps to greatly increase the number of decisions for divorce (Lopez and Munoz, 1980; Muñoz Vásquez, 1980). Acosta-Belen (1980), writing about Rene Marques's well-known story "*En la Popa hay un Cuerpo Reclinado*" (In the Stern There is a Corpse), gives a wonderful summary of the anti-feminism espoused by this famous author. Marques viewed North American influence in Puerto Rico as producing a kind of matriarchal pattern "Anglo-Saxon style," which renders men ineffectual (Rodriguez Ramos, 1976). Marques's women are generally portrayed as "castrating"; they destroy men's ideals of existential fulfillment. "The protagonist expresses his frustration caused by women who, according to him, have always tried to pressure him, influence him and direct his life" (Acosta-Belen, 1980:144).

It is also a fact that women are increasingly reported as victims of marital abuse, including homicide. Some studies estimate that one out of two women will suffer abuse from lovers or husbands at some time during their lives (Gravas, 1986–1987). (I remember a male friend, then an official high in the criminal justice division of the San Juan government, trying to justify the brutal axe death of a woman by her estranged husband. The woman's mutilated body had been accidentally discovered in a shallow grave. He pointed out to me that her ex-husband harbored righteous anger because she had been sexually involved with another man after separating from him!)

The women we knew well (both in and out of the Project) expressed ambivalence over both their sexuality and their self-worth. Some years ago I read about a survey conducted in 1960 among middle-class, teenaged boys and girls, sixteen to nineteen years old, which sought to elicit gender-related values. It found that only 3 percent of these young women felt that women should "wear the pants in the family." Thirty-four percent said that many women wish they were men. Only 29 percent said that they felt it was better to be a woman than a man. This study group represents today's late-middle-aged women, many of whom are successful professionals. In a more recent study, Rivera Ramos (1985) notes that her female subjects, ages eighteen to forty-seven (most currently younger than those in the previously mentioned study), drawn from working and nonworking lower- and middle-class urban groups, perceived themselves as self-sufficient, independent, and assertive. However, they viewed Puerto Rican women in general as passive and dependent. To many observers, women appear strong, persevering, and achieving, but the women themselves often discuss how limited they are in power and how strongly socially curtailed they are from being able to behave aggressively or even assertively.

As Christensen (1979) points out, gender-associated roles of women, as contrasted with those of men, are more narrowly constructed with regard to socially approved behavior. A girl (even as an infant) encounters restrictions in dress, freedom to move around, language usage, and sociality. In many open but also covert ways women acknowledge and complain about their lack of empowerment. They also seem to have internalized some ambivalence toward their destinies as mothers, subtly focused around their reproductive organs.

We noted that these views on women affected the health professionals and the Spiritist healers in different ways. The health professionals, including the medical doctors, have entered an opening in traditionally male-dominated professions at a time when health care services are expanding and admitting more women to their ranks. Because women in Puerto Rico in the past three decades have been more attracted to higher education than men, additional vocational opportunities have opened up for women, adding to the traditional "female professions" of teaching, social work, and nursing.

As older women, most of the Spiritists had not enjoyed higher education but had taken advantage of opportunities to fill quasi-institutionalized roles outside the economic system, available to persons who are retired from wage earning or family caretaking tasks. We observed that it is unusual for women to be recognized as powerful or important in these voluntary societal roles. Even professional women generally occupy middle-range jobs that support the institutions of which they are a part. And we knew many women *Espiritistas* who supported male presidents of the *centros* they (the women) actually organized and where they carried out the major healing work. (However, some others did direct their own *centros.*) Most of the healers who participated in the Project occupied subordinate social positions. They alternated between roles in families and jobs in institutions—which they faithfully and responsibly served, but never controlled.

In addition, we observed that the situation of women as healers in and of itself held several potential dangers. These dangers relate to the subtly articulated and covert attitudes about womanhood that many women seem to have taken as their own—however ambivalently—and feelings about their selves as female, especially regarding the culturally patterned (although highly individualized) experience of their bodies (see also Thompson, 1985). The dangers are linked to difficulties that arise out of the practice of healing. Spiritists express these dangers as allusions to the contagion of the illnesses they treat and fears of witchcraft (*trabajos malos*). They are also expressed through the deep frustration and "burnout" that health professionals and doctors frequently discuss. Spiritists, in particular, because they regularly enter into nonordinary states of consciousness with strange and distorted body movements in order to act as vehicles for healing forces, are regarded by many men and some women as possessing a perverse kind of power that could also be used to harm. Each of these three sources of problems for women healers—the paradoxical attitudes of men, women's ambivalence about their self-worth as women, and dangers that inhere to the healing role (especially for women)—will be described in detail in this chapter. Although these problem sources are briefly mentioned elsewhere, here I will try to weave together their separate strands of influence on the painful underside of the joy of healing.

The Feminine Eternally on Trial

Ortner's well-known paper (1974) asserts that women are universally perceived as closer to "nature" than to "culture" through their reproductive functions, social roles, and psychology. She sees woman's gender-determined roles as considered by most societies "to be at a lower order of the cultural process than man's" (1974:73). We observed that in Puerto Rico, women are often perceived by both men and women as subversive of the established order, for instance when they are feared for performing witchcraft or for being out of control in emotional, "hysterical" outbursts, but especially when they are seen as transgressing sexual mores. Yet at the very same time women are thought of as close to the divine because of their creative and restorative functions, both as mothers and as analogues for the suffering, sainted Mother of God. It is true that sometimes men are said to be responsible for witchcraft, and men occasionally flout sexual mores. However, men's behavior is more often overlooked and seems to bring about less serious consequences than women's.

In discussing Ortner's ideas, we decided that "nature" needs to be defined within a particular cultural context if we are to accept Ortner's formulation. In Puerto Rico "nature" is the raw, unsocialized, undomesticated, instinctual side of human being to which all are capable of succumbing. This aspect of one's being needs to be continually controlled in order to fulfill valued social requirements for conduct. But women are considered more able to manifest nature, perhaps because their reproductive and mothering roles are highly valued and thought of as "natural." One might say that women attract a projected distrust of the feminine, because both men and women seem to fear that the dependable, caring feminine way of being and behaving will fall out of its expected and forever-hoped-for place of ordered virtue and unlimited nurturance. The best of mothers inadvertently, or even consciously, inflicts pain from time to time and suffers from fear of doing so—in Puerto Rico as elsewhere.

Daughters are more aware of their mothers' falls from grace because early in life they perceive their mothers as models. They are aware that their mothers have the fatal flaw of covertly desiring the caring and consideration that mothers so poignantly fail to receive but so generously give. Mothers generally teach their daughters or model for them that they can never expect nurturance to continue beyond childhood. Sons are sought and groomed by women partly to satisfy their own emotional needs. Thus the nurturance of boys and of men is a continuous, almost seamless pattern while that of girls and women is discontinuous and erratic.

This dual-sided perspective on the feminine, that women possess the potential for being both very good and very bad at same time, is a contradiction inherent in nurturing activities, even those not directly associated with mothering. The woman-as-healer occupies an especially ambiguous place in a society plagued by widespread psychological ambivalence toward traditional healers (most of whom are women), whose practices are typified (as we have seen) by dealings with spirits, who are either very protective or very harmful. The woman-as-healer may be held in awe for her abilities, but she is also feared. This may be true for all shamanic-type healers (Peters and Price-Williams, 1980; Kakar, 1982), but male healers in most societies do not usually bring contradiction and ambivalence about their gender to their healer roles, even if these same roles visit this type of ambivalence on the male healer. Males are not seen as socially marginal or inferior before they become healers (although they may be viewed that way subsequently—in Puerto Rico and elsewhere), nor did the men in our project report that they became healers as an attempt to equalize or better their gender-determined social positions (Bourguignon, 1975; Lewis, 1971).

Although the Project was over when I read Cixous and Clement's description of the "sorceress" (which is used as a synonym for a role of women), there was instant recognition. These authors pair sorceress with another, more recent synonym, "hysteric." Both descriptions show the feminine to be "ambiguous, antiestablishment, and conservative"—at the same time. The sorceress is "able to dream nature and therefore conceive it. The hysteric, whose body is transformed into a theater for forgotten scenes, relives the past, bearing witness to a lost childhood that survives in suffering" (1986:5). Stories of women in either of these two roles illustrate the plight of those who passively do not conform but who nevertheless act out rebellious motives.

The "sorceress" and "hysteric" represent extremes, perhaps caricatures, of the two social roles described in this book—"healers" and "patients/clients." I suggest, however, that describing women as feared sorceresses or troubled hysterics has a ring of truth; in a sense these descriptions illuminate the predominant means by which Puerto Rican (and other) women attempt to deal with problems inherent in their role- and gender-defined fates by not overtly challenging either the domestic or the public power that men hold so tightly.

Witchcraft

Perhaps only the traditional healers, the *Espiritistas*, can be viewed through the "sorceress" lens as the inheritors and acquisitors of an anomalous social role, one outside the symbolic and structural order of ordinary social life. Their intense relationships with spirits—especially their flamboyant possessions—their intimacy with pain and suffering, and their compelling nurturing attitudes toward everyone, make them suspect. Although all the *Espiritistas* I know disavow spirit work that would harm rather than heal, a widespread underlying fear of their special kind of power lends itself to thoughts about, and direct accusations of their being, witches (*brujas*). Stories of going to spirit workers to prepare a harmful "work" or charm (*trabajo malo, hechizo, magia negra, dano*) are not uncommon. Some *Espiritistas* are reputed to be able to "revoke" the harmful "work," which can include turning it back onto its originator. Yet none of the healers who participated in our seminars identified herself as a witch or worked at preparing *trabajos*. Moreover, many explicitly harangued clients who reported that they had sought (or bought) a "spell" (*hechizo*). At one session, Doña Tati vehemently told her client:

> Well, look, that *Espiritista* did not help you. This class of *Espiritista* doesn't help anyone. Because there is no better spell than if you think that they had done something. What the *Espiritista* should do is help the person. There are very many classes of traditional healers who believe in [bad] works and spells, and one medium can make a fool out of [*embabucar*] the other. Then, instead of helping the person, what they do is unhelpful [*desayuda*] because they are augmenting evil. Our spiritual mission is divine. You must extract yourself, stop thinking about *trabajos* and things that don't exist.

We observed many persons who were suffering from spells arranged by others who wished them ill and who came to the *centros* for help in countering the "bad work." They were treated spiritually in the usual ways; however, there was more emphasis on acquiring spirit protection (Harwood, 1977). The general ideological message of most *Espiritistas* is that evil does not exist except in the belief of those persons who feel attacked. *Espiritistas* explained that distressed spirits (who have died an untimely or violent death or who desire vengeance because of a hurt inflicted by the client in a past life relationship) unwittingly inflict harm, and they can be convinced not to do so. Although it is recognized that a few spirit mediums do arrange evil spells, they are excluded from the informal fraternity of *Espiritistas* and are generally regarded as misguided, unwise individuals who do not really intend evil. The sensitive observer rather quickly becomes aware of the intense affect projected by most *Espiritistas* in attempts to dissociate themselves from "ignorant, superstitious persons" who do not follow the sacred mandate to align oneself only with forces of "light." The energy expended in the effort to avoid being identified as a worker of "black magic" or as a "witch" speaks to an ever-present fear of social disapproval (and even stigma) that is openly preached from many pulpits, particularly by Catholic priests and fundamentalist ministers. And although I know of no cases involving Spiritist practices that have received attention from law enforcement agencies in the past twenty years, it is well known that some medical doctors criticize Spiritist practices (even though a minority of medical doctors are believers and a few are also *Espiritistas*). Fear of legal sanctions seems to have motivated the division of labor by Spiritists into *causa material* and *causa espiritual*, and the consistent referral of the *material* cases to medical doctors.

The skepticism shown by Spiritist mediums is not shared by persons who believe their illnesses are the results of *hechizos*, or black magic. Both men and women report illness histories with one or more *trabajos* as the cause of particular episodes or symptoms. For example, an elderly man who presented to a medical clinic said, "They did a work against me in 1958 in Ponce. I was in the hospital for one month. I was swollen, my armpits didn't function. In '65 they did another work: a scaly rash came out my hands, I felt desperate and nervous. I felt like my hands had contracted [shrunk]. In '66 a rash came out on my neck. Because of this I don't trust anyone."

Hilda, a woman of thirty-seven years and a patient in day care at a mental health center, reported that for more than two years she had felt "dead in life," had difficulty sleeping, and had experienced a number of "delusions" about bodily symptoms, especially that her genitals itched and felt as if they were disintegrating. She said that all her problems were her husband's fault. They quarreled a great deal, and he took her to *centros* where *Espiritistas* "worked with plants." Hilda felt this work to be harmful rather than healing, causing her both emotional and physical problems.

At the case review session where Hilda was presented, the psychologist explained that her patient's symptoms were the result of delusions, expressions of her anxieties about her husband. The *Espiritistas*, in contrast, viewed the symptoms as caused by spirits, because she was in "development." Other therapists felt that Hilda was creating the symptoms to get out of her marriage but had now convinced herself that they were real. We commented upon the lack of certainty in both the therapists' and the Spiritists' explanations of the "real" reason for Hilda's symptoms.

Later we discussed our observation that when confronted with someone who believed in witchcraft, even health professionals trained in scientific explanations of illness causality were ambivalent about denying the existence of witchcraft. Perhaps even more important is the fact that many *Espiritistas* expressed their suspicions that other spirit mediums with whom they were not associated did arrange harmful spells. These views served to reinforce the suspicions of the therapists and doctors who participated in the Project. For example, one doctor reported her confusion when a seriously ill young woman, who had worked as a medium for two years, said she was "covered by a white mantle because she had been the target of many evil works."

The following account, given by a medical doctor regarding a patient concerned with the continuing illness of her infant son—conceived out of wedlock with a married man—illustrates how male/female relations, especially extramarital relations, frequently generate conflict that leads to accusations (or use) of witchcraft. "The mother says that the wife of the baby's father is a person who frequently goes to *Espiritistas*, and one threw something in front of the patio of her house, according to the neighbors. After this the baby suffered a severe fever." Although this young woman also told her doctor that she had gone with a relative to see an *Espiritista* when her child had suffered an earlier illness, and even said that she had found a successful cure, she claimed not to believe in Spiritism. But she did believe in the possibility that the child's current illness had been been caused by an evil spell bought by her rival.

A number of cases are described by Harwood (1977) of Puerto Ricans in New York where, as in other U.S. communities, witchcraft beliefs may be even more common than in Puerto Rico. What is important is the way belief in witchcraft exacerbates conflicts among women (and between women and men), especially over that important aspect of women's lives that does most to validate feelings of self-worth—good mothering. The *Espiritistas*, of whom two-thirds to three-fourths are women, are sometimes seen as the facilitators, if not the causes, of bad works, because they have power to manipulate agencies beyond the control of other persons. These accusations resonate with those of persons projecting the identity of "sorceress" onto *Espiritistas*. When a child is attacked by illness and the agent of the attack is a woman (as is usually the case), an image of the dark, Medea-like underside of the feminine emerges. In my observations, I found this image is so feared that it is rarely acknowledged as a personal feeling.

Illness and Contagion

We considered the idea that because retrospective accounts are so subject to selective perception, it is impossible to say whether women healers actually experienced more severe illness when young or whether they simply have more vivid memories of illness because they were more impressed with their negative experiences. An attempt to measure the current levels and types of complaints was made by asking the healers to respond to the Cornell Medical Index, a list of 195 current and chronic complaints and past illnesses. The results confirmed some of our speculations about the higher prevalence of illness in these women. In terms of overall frequency of positive responses, their mean scores were higher than those considered standard for U.S. populations.[1] On one scale Spiritists scored a significant difference as compared with other groups of healers; they reported more serious childhood and adult illnesses as well as current and past extremes of weight. Spiritists also reported more complaints on three other scales—somatic and behavioral complaints related to emotional distress, interpersonal sensitivity, and nervousness—as compared with therapists and doctors. Therapists' and doctors' mean scores on another three scales—irritable and angry responses, feelings of fatigue, and skin problems—showed a trend of being higher than those of Spiritists.

However, there are almost no overall differences between types of women healers in their self-reports of current illness complaints. And even the one significant finding, of more childhood and chronic illness in Spiritists, is not significant when age is statistically controlled. Compared with a community sample of housewives in a lower-middle-class housing development in Puerto Rico, the mean positive responses of healers across types were somewhat lower than the 46.4 for the housewives (Koss, 1974). The mean total number of complaints for the three groups of healers were: Spiritists, 29.25; mental health workers, 22.12; and doctors, 23.28—not significantly different. These means are only a bit lower than the general criterion of 30 positive responses used to indicate serious emotional disorder in U.S. samples. This can be accounted for by the very frequent use of the body in idioms of distress. Individual responses of women in each of the healer groups ranged from seven to ninety-one complaints for Spiritists, one to sixty-nine complaints for therapists, and two to fifty-nine complaints for medical doctors. This wide range in individual responses to the Cornell Medical Index makes comparison difficult. Fourteen healers in all three groups gave positive answers to thirty or more items on the index; thus some of the healers were near or above the means (73.7 and 71.74) for small samples of mental health patients in Puerto Rico and New York. It seems important to ask why some women healers experience (or express) so much distress.

It has been suggested by one anthropologist that some women in the Mediterranean tradition and their descendants in Latin America and the Caribbean cope with malaise and dysphoric affect through a public "rhetoric of complaint" that brings them respect because of their extensive experience with illness and problems (Gaines and Farmer, 1986). Although Spiritists are generally known (or more accurately, sensed) to have had and overcome severe distress, they rarely talked about it unless asked (as we did in our interviews). Mental health workers and doctors seemed reluctant to complain, even when asked about their own illnesses and problems. They preferred not to be seen as vulnerable or wounded. This defense against feelings of malaise and distress can lead to problems that I will describe later. In general, the woman who is stoical and in charge of her life is an ideal of Puerto Rican womanhood. For Spiritists she is personified by Amalia Domingo Soler, one of the founders of the movement in Spain. Amalia, though blind and ill most of her life, never flagged in her duty to care for her elderly mother or help others. There is a sense of martyrdom and self-sacrifice in this ideal picture, but it does not praise the woman who "cries" or complains excessively.

One important reason for the Spiritist healers' experiencing high levels of distress may be an identification with the pains and problems of clients and patients. In Chapter 4 I described how Spiritist healers "capture" or form the symptoms of their clients in their own bodies as a routine aspect of healing rituals. Recent discussions in some psychoanalytic circles of the importance of understanding countertransference reactions in the analyst are of interest here (Samuels, 1985). In contrast to classical views that countertransference reactions in the analyst should be suppressed or dealt with apart from patients, there is now more recognition of the analyst's total emotional involvement in his or her relationship with a patient, especially on the unconscious level. However, although some analysts advocate that their feelings should be taken into account in interpreting the therapeutic process, they also feel that these feelings should not be talked about within the therapeutic session. A more extreme view is that both patient and analyst are equally part of the therapeutic interactional field, and that the psychoanalyst's contribution is as important as that of the patient (Langs, 1978). In this process, as described by Langs, the analyst is trying to put something of his own psyche, in relation to the patient's problem, into the patient. The patient in turn places his or her distress into the analyst's mind. This is described as so disturbing and upsetting an experience that it cannot be ignored by the analyst. Thus the analyst is able to gain special access to the patient's inner state and has a more compelling (one could say intimate) motivation to work on the patient's distress because the work is done within both the analyst's and the patient's psyches.

The dynamic process of identification between Spiritist healer and client has a parallel motive. However, it is, at least at first, a largely nonverbal interchange of feelings and emotions, mediated by spiritual currents (*flúidos; corrientes magnéticos*). As it proceeds, both directness and metaphor are added to communications between Spiritist and client in terms of specific probes about the client's condition and circumstances and identification of the spirits molesting or supporting her. As described earlier, spirits perceived and experienced as "stuck onto" the client register their pain or distressing emotions inside the healer. At first the healer only "sees" into the spirit world to describe her client's problems (*videncias*). (She is protected by her principal spirit guide, who stands behind her while she works at the table.) But gradually the spirit invades the healer's body-consciousness (*plasmar*), and she reports feeling exactly what her client feels. The identity of the spirit and how it is causing the client's state then become evident, and the healer or another medium will feel able (that is, protected and strong enough) to "call" the spirit *causa* into her body. Through this ritual vehicle, the harmful, backward, unenlightened spirit can speak. This kind of healing transaction depends upon the healer being physically and psychically open to dangerous and negative affects stemming from the client's illness or malaise.

Thus the Spiritist healer consciously accepts a state of increased vulnerability in order to carry out healing practices. The strength of her personal life force—her resistance and power to deal with illness and severe distress—is continually on the line. It is at this juncture in the healing ritual and during encounters and consultations outside the *centro* that contagion of clients' malaise is a definite possibility. Yet the notion of contagion is not straightforward as in the sense of communication of infection; it refers more to the idea that the healer may already be in a weakened state (due to "material" illness or problems that she has recently suffered or to disturbances in relations with one or more of her spirit guides or to ethical problems in her life). She will be further weakened to the extent that she will show physical or psychological effects. The concept that I have labeled "contagion" is illustrated by Spiritists' reports of fear of harmful effects on the healer through contact with a client who carries extremely negative vibrations (because she is inevitably plagued by numerous low or backward spirits). This was echoed in the comments of the mental health workers, who felt "depressed" or "nervous" after a full day with severely mentally ill patients.

The Spiritists described the presence of *guías* in positive terms, even as extremely pleasant, with moods and feelings of "contentment," "security," "warmth," "relaxation," and "peacefulness." However, they made clear that the experience of one's body being entered by any spirit is uncomfortable and strange, especially when one is inexperienced. Many said that spirits are felt to enter through the top of the head (they point to a place close to where the pineal gland and the centroencephalon are located). Some mediums described this sensation as an "explosion" in the brain (see also Nuñez Molina, 1987); others simply talked about a kind of headache and sensations of heaviness at the base of the skull. The general process of being "possessed" by a spirit is sometimes described as a feeling of great fullness and discomfort; the body feels as if under increasing pressure until the spirit-energy obtains a release and the spirit is "passed" by the medium. The experience of *videncias* or of *causa* spirits is said to be extremely uncomfortable and even painful. The medium may feel "tired," "tense," very "nervous," and fearful. There is almost always a disagreeable sensation of heat; sometimes hot and cold sensations alternate. Mediums said they feel their blood pressure rising, and sometimes they experience a buzzing sound in their ears. Several mediums mentioned that their heart rates accelerate; they can hear their hearts beating loudly. Everyone reported feeling subject to the alien will of the spirit possessing them. They related that they may hear the spirit speaking but always feel dissociated from the voice. One medium, describing her experience, said, "One continues saying things that in truth I don't know where they come from; and even when I am conscious, that is, I hear everything around me, I feel fearful, subconsciously, that someone will ask me something. But I know that the force (*móvil*) that makes me speak answers correctly."

The general conception that seemed to us to unite these descriptions of visionary and spirit-possession experiences was that of fluidity or flexibility in consciousness of self as the subject of experience. We observed that possession-trance is largely a feminine activity in Spiritism (there are approximately three to four women *Espiritistas* to every man, and relatively few men become possessed). It is therefore important to examine how women feel about their bodies in the context of healing work. We reflected upon the observation that idioms often used to describe the experience of possession-trance seem to analogize it with negative sexual experiences. Several healers agreed that possession by a *causa* spirit felt like "rape." Others talked about the spirit "penetrating" their bodies. The sensations of being "filled up" by the spirit, of "heat" experienced "deep in the body" contribute to the sense that the possessed medium feels dominated, oppressed by a foreign force personified (for the sake of description) as an external being.

However, we could not say that these descriptions referred in a symbolic way to sexuality per se. Consonant with traditional taboos about the subject, especially in mixed groups, sexual intercourse is almost always referred to obliquely in either spirit or direct communications both within and without the ritual sessions. When spirit mediums do refer to sexual intercourse it is usually expressed by euphemisms, such as "going to bed" or "marital relations." And there is the ever-present, underlying assumption that a husband has a legitimate right to direct and control his mate's sexuality. (We thought that the experience of possession-trance is analogous to relations with men in general: it is thought of as inevitable, inescapable, and requiring submission.) We discussed the notion that both spirit-healer and male-female relationships are felt to be both highly desirable and very difficult and dangerous—another facet of the ambivalence that characterizes women's lives and thoughts.[2]

The sensations of flexibility and fluidity that mediums report in the experience of consciousness during healing work can perhaps be thought of as necessary to the relationship between healer and client with regard to countertransference as a therapeutic process. Spiritist healing insists upon an "embodied countertransference," that is, the embodiment of a "physical, actual, material, sensual expression" in the healer of something in his (or her) client's inner world (Samuels, 1985:52). This may be appreciated in the following account of a novice medium's initial experience of a client.

> I went with Doña Sara to help a paralyzed woman. I was privately feeling very sorry for her. When I saw her I felt a creeping heaviness in my arm. It went up and then down my spine, stopping in the middle. I then got the same feeling in my legs, in one more than the other. Then I could no longer move my legs. The woman said it came on in just that way during four days. She had never told anyone that before. Doña Sara said that you have to talk about it for the feelings to leave. As soon as I spoke about my feelings, they went away and I felt calm.

The *embodiment* of a patient's feelings is rarely mentioned by mental health workers or doctors. However, deep empathy was evinced, as in the case of Mili, a psychiatric social worker. After describing the conflict in her childhood home because her father drank and caroused with women (and neighbors continually informed her mother of his activities), she said, "Because of this experience, I understand more about a child when he comes here hurt by family problems. I can get to him (*llegar*) more easily." We frequently noted that, despite the lack of direct references to countertransference effects in their descriptions of work with patients, many of the mental health professionals talked about fears that clients would become too dependent upon them. In response to this fear they spaced therapy sessions to avoid what they perceived as "overdependence" in certain clients. It seemed that they were very willing to nurture their clients, although in limited ways. Most therapists were clearly not willing to feel uncomfortable about or "take on" clients' problems. The rhetoric of "overdependence" seemed to us to be a defense against what we labeled "contagion," that is, becoming like a patient.

The doctors, on the other hand, felt that the degree of social distance considered appropriate between patients and physicians frequently lead physicians to be "rude" (literally to lack "culture") and ignorant of patients' ideas and feelings. These young women advocated a relationship of *confianza* (mutual trust). But in our view their comments spoke also to a defense against "contagion"; they practiced avoidance of personal involvement. Their case write-ups (and those of the male doctors) described patients only superficially (apart from physical problems) and only occasionally recorded a patient's own concerns about the illness.

We encountered a deep feeling among mental health workers, although rarely verbalized directly, of fear of becoming emotionally disordered themselves. As mentioned earlier, both they and the doctors were very aware of emotional problems and mental illness within their immediate and extended families. They also readily acknowledged some of their own past and present problems. The difficulties of becoming a patient when one is a healer and expected to be invulnerable (or immune) to severe emotional disturbance are illustrated in the following account of attempted suicide. This occurred when the mental health worker was participating in the Project.

> Rosa, divorced, with five children, was having difficulties with her live-in boyfriend (who was in treatment at the mental health center). In addition, she felt overwhelmed at times and frustrated in her job. Having had experience with *Espiritistas* through her mother's prolonged mental illness, she became friendly with two Spiritist participants who lived in her hometown. She said, "One night I was feeling OK, but I took some pills (Estrafon) and sat on the bed next to my boyfriend; he said I was acting strangely. I asked for a Mellaril [thioridazine] and promised to cut it in quarters, but I took it all and went to sleep. The next morning I awakened and my boyfriend was going to Caguas [a nearby town]. I insisted on going with him even though he said I should stay home and rest. On the way I dropped over—asleep. He took me to the hospital [the health center]; I was unconscious. They pumped my stomach, but the pills weren't harmful and I was all right. Then the intern called my friends, the *Espiritistas*, and I went home with them.[3] At the end of the week they took me to a session and rid me of three *causas* [illness causing spirits]."

Rosa apparently felt uncertain about whether her colleagues should know about her emotional problems. She called a meeting of several whom she felt would "understand." There she played an audiotape of the Spiritist session in which she had been treated, but she did not identify herself as the client. It seemed clear to us that she felt compelled to tell her colleagues about herself, however indirectly this was accomplished. Later we heard gossip that her participation in the Spiritist session was recognized. To those few friends whom she told about the incident, she maintained that she had been "obsessed" by spirits and was completely unaware of her actions on the days she overdosed.[4]

Coping with Contagion

When asked how long *causa* spirits affect a medium-healer who allows herself to become possessed by them, the general opinion was that it depends on the type of *causa*. One *Espiritista* said that a "drug or liquor" *causa* may affect her for several days before "her stomach can accept food." She "needs to pray in order to send the badness into the ether." The prescribed remedy during a session is an exorcistic cleansing; the *guía* presiding over the healer's "work" at the table "cleans" the medium's body so that it feels "lighter," "relieved," and "more relaxed." One woman said that she felt "happier" and "optimistic" after the cleansing. It seems almost impossible to avoid "taking the *causa*" into one's body once a relationship with a "principal *guía*" is consolidated. A medium-healer said, for example, "If I don't manifest the sick spirit, my *guía* will punish me."

By working at the table as a group that usually includes mediums who have "developed" under the guidance of the president or have aligned themselves with her, Spiritist healers feel better protected against the contagion of clients' distress. They all generally agree that this is the only safe way to work. Although they may hold individual consultations, they regularly recommended that clients attend the next scheduled *centro* meeting. The president's principal protector-guide spirit presides over all the work at the *centro* and will come to the rescue of a medium who is having difficulty passing a spirit. Most mediums will not work during times when the spiritual environment is charged, such as during Christmas or Holy Week; they also stop working when ill—if the condition is interpreted as spirit-caused.

I noted some time ago that qualities inherent in the organization and dynamics of these cult groups eventually serve to undermine their method of "group protection" and even endanger the equilibrium individuals have achieved through development as healers (Koss, 1977). The reader may recall the description in Chapter 3 of how mediums are recruited. Once diagnosed as "in development," if they express the wish to become mediums, they will be encouraged to sit at or very near the table. They assume a quasi-apprenticeship role in relation to the president of the *centro*, with whom they usually form a close relationship of dependence and support (Koss, 1975). In this way a *centro's* leader and founder expands the work she directs and acquires greater status as a healer. Not only is the president responsible for the protection of all the mediums when they are possessed by *causa* spirits, and the final judge of the accuracy of the *videncias*, but she is also considered the most advanced spirit worker. Her status is enhanced by her reputation as an effective vehicle for the spirits. The more successful the cures she effects, the better her reputation and the greater the number of mediums she can attract to her table. The *centro* is usually known by her name (unless it is an organized *templo*, or "school," such as one that follows the teachings of Joaquin Trincado, an Argentinian disciple of Kardec). Her fame is augmented by the work of her mediums, because she is known to preside over all that takes place at the table.

Although there is no formal hierarchy beyond a president, mediums may acquire reputations as effective healers in their own rights. Sooner or later they begin to seek autonomy with regard to validating their own experiences of spirits, which presents a problem for the president of the *centro*, who is considered to "know" more than her disciples. Some who challenge the president's authority may decide to leave the group and establish their own *centros*. At times, rather distressing conflicts disturb the close-knit, quasi-familial ambience of the *centros'* groups of mediums and followers. Because there is no formal organization and each *centro* is an individual cult group, there are no regulations or understandings that govern the new *centros* that split off from the mother groups. They do not relate as daughter groups by acknowledging their ties and subordination to the *centros* where their leaders were novitiate mediums. Moreover, their separations most commonly result from disagreements over clients or points of ideology, because there are no specified ways to deal with conflicts in interpretations of the meanings or behavior of spirits.

We observed that these dynamics created a dangerous paradox both for the leader of a *centro* and for the mediums she recruits. The personal transformations that women undergo when they become mediums in part depend on the supportive environment offered by their presidents and other mediums. Interpersonal conflict can destroy the benefits offered by the intimacy and support a medium enjoys within the inner circle of the *centro* and can thus threaten her newly found adjustment. Her choice is to withdraw from the group or attempt to organize a *centro* of her own—if she can attract other mediums to work at her side. These interpersonal dynamics are often at the bottom of accusations of witchcraft, which are frequently expressions of the fear that very intimate knowledge about a medium's *guías* will be bantered about in other *centros*. This kind of knowledge makes attacks at a distance, using "bad works," a definite possibility. The core of the medium's consciousness of self can then be breached, and depending on the strength of her new adjustment to life, she can again be threatened with illness.

Mediums sometimes say that the more developed they are, the more "immune" they are to illnesses of clients. For example, one medium commented about her dealings with a client suffering from tuberculosis.

> It [immunity] has come about by developing through spiritual evolution and the dematerialization [sic] of the soul during the reincarnations. I have dealt with tuberculosis an infinity of times; I have been in contact with patients with TB; I have never caught the disease. Why? Because I have in my body-soul an immunity that I have acquired through reincarnations, that is able to defend me against this illness; but it may be that you do not have that quality.

However, we were often told by mediums that development presents its own problems. Mediums have to work hard to satisfy the demands of some of their *guías*, such as that they should not marry or should erect an altar for daily worship. We speculated that these demands parallel a person's reckoning with her superego (to use a psychological analogy). Both personal salvation and prestige in the cult group develop in a linear fashion. Progress is conceived as moving upward toward the high moral ideals personified in the behavior of the saints. The journey "upward" is beset by bad thoughts as well as bad works that must be overcome; difficulties arise both within and without. As a medium becomes more adept at communicating with the spirit world and effecting cures on behalf of clients, the sources of danger to her person multiply because she is constantly revealing aspects of her "protections" in the service of her work at the table and in the training of other mediums. Moreover, she has to consistently show her "strength" to be able to protect other mediums who work at her table. In sum, the more famous a Spiritist medium becomes, the more self-sufficient she is supposed to be; but at the same time, there is a greater possibility of contagion and a greater likelihood that "bad works" will be directed at her or at her mediums. She also suffers greater exposure to strong, illness-causing bad spirits as clients with more serious problems seek her out. The president's "progress" thus becomes a matter of renouncing dependency on all but her personal spirit guides. What is her recourse in times of serious illness or other crises?

This dilemma became quite evident when, some years after the Project ended, Doña Aida (one of our principal participants) suffered a stroke. Although physically incapacitated and confined to a wheel chair, she was alert and as spiritually adept as ever. However, when she sought to resume her work as president of her *centro*, her mediums began to question her "protection" and spiritual strength. They told us that so serious an illness was perceived by them as vulnerability rather than the desired quality (especially for a leading medium) of immunity, a quality necessary to protect them against the effects of illness-causing spirits. Although Doña Aida continued to work on a reduced schedule, her own faith in her protections had been seriously shaken. She was not supported by her own mediums, who felt she should retire. Her only supporter at the time was a medium from another *centro*, whom she came to know through the Project and whose center dissolved because of conflict. This medium, although an outsider to Doña Aida's *centro*, had assisted Doña Aida on occasion. We heard her tell the mediums that the "body is unimportant" in spirit work. She insisted that Doña Aida still had deep and important spirit powers but was forced to adapt to her condition and regain her former level of self-confidence.

General Observations on the Problems of Women as Healers

A number of writers have described the many ways in which women in all societies are excluded from participating in realms that represent the greatest power (Ortner, 1974; La Fontaine, 1981; Littlewood and Lipsedge, 1987). Whether by custom or by law, an ideology focused on men's concerns and experiences is the basic tool of exclusion. In turn, women's realms are commonly structured by perceptions of their anatomy and physiology. As in preindustrial societies in general, women in Puerto Rico are expected to marry and have children. These goals are considered the "natural" ones for women and so important that they must be "protected" while acquiring professional status. Such views may be overtly or covertly regarded with ambivalence by many women, yet women seem continually to collude in the achievement of this male-oriented design. In this way, those who possess female reproductive physiology are set up to think of themselves as they are regarded—as weak, passive, dependent, and, especially, unempowered.

The ironic adjunct to the situation of Puerto Rican women is that so many Puerto Rican men fail to meet the responsibilities assigned to them as women's "protectors." This poses a serious dilemma; women are expected to (and do) subordinate their self-interests to those of their families and the commonweal. There are many social and economic reasons for men's failures, but regardless of the reasons, the result is that the subordination of women's self-interests to those of family and society is all the more necessary. First, because men derive a good deal of status from having offspring and expect women to fulfill this need; and second, because men hardly suffer (at least at present) for their failure to perform responsibly as husbands and fathers. In fact, the current ideology for men says that they can hardly be expected to consistently fulfill their male obligations.

We know that such formulations cannot be stated in a categorical way because many cases contrary to these observations could be cited. Yet examples, such as the case of Ida, are becoming increasingly common.

> Ida's mother and father were generally uncommunicative. They never spoke about sexual matters or emotional ones either. At nine years of age Ida was sent to live, temporarily, with her father's sister and her husband. Ida's aunt was the person who explained things to her when she reached *menarche* and was kinder to her than her own mother was. Her aunt's husband seemed interested in her as well and took to visiting her in her room late at night. Ida loved the affection he showed her, and his "playing" led to sexual intercourse. She only told her aunt about it when she was fourteen years old; two years later she became pregnant with her uncle's child. She continued to have sexual relations with her uncle because she felt no one else would marry her. He rarely helped her financially, but her aunt, who was childless, sent money even when they moved to the States. The aunt adopted Ida's oldest boy, and although she threatened divorce, stayed with her husband even though he ran around with several women in New York. She knew that he continued to drink and continued to have sexual relations with Ida (he fathered two more children with her). Ida felt trapped by the relationship and never again was intimate with another man. She finally stopped the thirty-two-year relationship some five years ago when she joined a fundamentalist church.

We discussed Ardener's work (1978), in which he suggests that the sexes can "pollute" each other when there is a perceived important difference between a male model for behavior and an opposing model that women force men to consider. By showing consistent responsibility toward her family and husband, a woman is behaving in a way very different from that of many men in Puerto Rico, who are considered to be "free spirits" by nature. Moreover, the role of healer fills out the feminine model in ways clearly at variance with the male model. By becoming healers women can acquire power through a combination of prestigious interpersonal relations and responsible nurturance. These attributes are also much desired by men but resented when women possess them. This is so because healer roles clearly represent aspects of feminine power (such as nurturance) that cannot be subordinated to the interests of men.

Notes

1. See also Garrison, 1977a, and Finkler, 1985, for similar findings among Puerto Ricans in New York and Mexicans in the Yucatán, especially among women.

2. See Littlewood and Lipsedge (1987) for a detailed analysis of this theme.

3. This doctor was also a project participant and responded to Rosa's plea that she would lose her job if her colleagues at the mental health center heard about her attempted suicide. He instead called the Spiritists (whom he also knew) because he felt they would attend to her immediately and with more concern than she would receive from emergency services at the mental health center.

4. A number of mental health professionals and medical doctors who participated in the Project consulted the *Espiritistas* for their own problems once they knew the *Espiritistas* personally (the reverse was also true, but the Spiritists consulted the mental health workers less frequently) (Koss, 1980).

6

Psychiatric Illness, Emotional Disorder, and Women's Experience

La locura de mi alma *no puede reclinarse,* *vive en lo inquieto,* *en lo desordenado,* *en el desequilibrio* *de las cosas dinámicas,* *en el silencio* *del libre pensador, que vive solo,* *en callado destierro.*	*The craziness of my soul* *cannot rest,* *it lives in the disquiet,* *disorder* *and disequilibrium* *of dynamic things,* *in the silence* *of the free thinker, who lives alone,* *in hushed exile.*

—Julia de Burgos, "Mi *Alma*"

Perspectives on Mental Disorder and Emotional Distress

Psychiatry labels severe emotional distress, impaired intellectual functioning, and maladaptive behavior as "mental" or "psychiatric" illness or disorder. Such illness is conceptualized as the expression of biologically based, internal, abnormal "mental" or central nervous system states. In contrast, Spiritist ideology explains physical and emotional distress and associated problems in living as individualized genres of spirit intervention related to or caused by inharmonious or immoral behavior in this or a past life. These contrasting explanations of prolonged disturbance in emotions and behavior lack a common denominator: Spiritists do not use a concept of "mind" to explain the cause of distress or disorder as do those trained in psychology or psychiatry. Instead they view "mind" as synonymous with "brain," a special place in the body where disturbances can occur. And we know that psychiatry denies and denigrates the existence of "spirits," which are the keys to causality and treatment for Spiritists.

These contrasting explanations of emotional distress and behaviorial disorder and the healing practices associated with them were the soil in which the Therapist-Spiritist Project seeded an interchange through a series of seminar programs based upon a clinical methodology that included peer teaching and modeling. The Project's programs were the vehicles for communicating ideas and knowledge about differing beliefs, guidelines, scientific knowledge, and ideology related to the diagnosis and treatment of emotional distress. But they also provided an excellent opportunity to collect data, not only on the healer-participants, but also on three opportunity samples of the patients and clients of core participants. The largest sample consisted of 1,769 patients and clients of healers during the month prior to, and the month following, their participation. A second sample consisted of one hundred new patients and clients in each year, who were interviewed while they awaited their first treatments at the clinics or *centros* of the core participants. A third sample consisted of all the cases presented at the case review sessions held each week during the seminar programs. (The general characteristics of patients and clients, both men and women, are given in Tables A.4 and A.5 in the Appendix.) With two exceptions (in preceding chapters), we describe only the cases and experiences of the women.

In this chapter, I first provide a brief overview of the prevalence and patterning of mental disorders in Puerto Rico summarized from published studies in psychiatric epidemiology. This is offered as background to an analysis of profiles of naturally occurring complaints, including the meanings of individual complaints and the patterns of experience associated with them. These complaints expressed how women as patients and clients of the healer-participants in the Project experienced emotional and cognitive distress and disorder. To arrive at the patterns and profiles, I used therapists' diagnoses, based upon the main psychiatric higher-rank diagnostic categories, as points of departure for the analyses of cases in order to understand which cases being treated by healers in different healing systems could be categorized as "mental illness" and which cases could be defined as less severe emotional or physical distress. Those patients and clients with cases of lesser severity, which were not included within the psychiatric diagnostic system, were sometimes treated by therapists and a few were seen by doctors in primary care clinics, but most went to Spiritist healers. The systematic construction of complaint profiles was based upon a statistical analysis of the largest sample of 779 cases of men and 990 cases of women. (The Appendix includes a description of the analytical methodology as well as tables that illustrate the profiles and their major dimensions.)

Psychiatric Illness Among Puerto Ricans

Some time ago Haberman (1976) investigated psychiatric symptoms among Puerto Ricans in New York and Puerto Rico using the twenty-two item screening instrument from the Midtown Manhattan Study. He found that people in an islandwide community sample from Puerto Rico gave positive responses more often than Puerto Ricans in two samples from the New York metropolitan area. It is of interest that women, people in the forty- to sixty-four-year age group, previously married people or those in common-law relationships, and people with less education or income reported significantly more psychiatric symptoms than their peers in the United States. Moreover, these scores were high as compared with U.S. response patterns, indicating the possibility of either a higher rate of impairment or a cultural pattern that favors the production of complaints. Haberman concluded in favor of the latter.

The most systematic and recent study of psychiatric illness in Puerto Rico is an extension of the Epidemiologic Catchment Area (ECA) program, which used the Diagnostic Interview Schedule (DIS), translated and adapted by Canino (Canino et al., 1987a; Canino et al., 1987b; Bravo et al., 1991).[1] This study examined a range of mental disorders, including affective (mood) disorders, anxiety, somatization and schizophrenic disorders, alcohol abuse, psychosexual dysfunction, and cognitive impairment. Excluding psychosexual dysfunction, a 28 percent lifetime prevalence rate was found for all disorders. The authors conclude that approximately 450,000 people in Puerto Rico met criteria for one or more psychiatric disorders over their lifetimes. Of particular interest is the finding that women had significantly higher lifetime prevalence rates of affective and phobic disorders and also of psychosexual dysfunction. Lifetime and six-month prevalence rates decreased with higher education; lifetime rates for anxiety disorders and alcohol abuse increased with age; and schizophrenic and somatization disorders were more prevalent between twenty-five and forty-four years of age.

The investigators note that these rates for mental disorders do not differ significantly from those reported for other ECA sites in the continental United States, with the exception of cognitive impairment and somatization disorder, both of which have higher rates in Puerto Rico. Somatization disorder, in particular, seems to have a very different expression in Puerto Rico where both men and women met the criteria, in contrast to other ECA sites where only women met the criteria.

Canino and her colleagues (1987a) note that these rates may be related to the findings of earlier studies in which Puerto Rican men and women tended to report a large number of symptoms in general, particularly somatic symptoms. These researchers point out problems of standardization when using another language and when measuring rates across very different cultural and social contexts (Bravo, 1991). However, they feel comfortable concluding that approximately the same numbers of Puerto Ricans suffer mental disorders as do persons in communities in the United States where other ECA studies have been carried out, such as St. Louis, Missouri; New Haven, Connecticut; and Baltimore, Maryland.

Studies of Higher-Rank Categories of Psychiatric Disorder: Depression and Anxiety

Hispanic women in populations in the United States consistently suffer between two and three times the number of depressive disorders as do Hispanic men (Vernon and Roberts, 1982; Frerichs et al., 1981; Wiessman and Klerman, 1977; Vega et al., 1984). In Puerto Rico the rate for women is four and one-half times greater that the rate for men. Among the various reasons given to explain why women are at high risk for depression, Canino and her colleagues (1987c) analyzed the factors of employment, marital status, and health status. They found that if previously married and in poor health, Puerto Rican women are at higher risk for depression than are men with the same characteristics. With regard to employment, Canino's findings were that married and employed women, and married and unemployed women are at about equal risk for depressive disorders. She points out that being a housewife is not as disvalued a status in Puerto Rico as in the United States and, in fact, women's work roles are not as important as their roles as mothers and wives. However, she also notes that these factors do not entirely account for the high prevalence of depression among women, which requires a somewhat different type of analysis than that offered by psychiatric epidemiology.

Torres-Matrullo (1982), studying mainland Puerto Rican women, highlights social and psychological aspects of women's roles as contributing factors in their depression. She lists "depressogenic cognitions," such as prohibition of anger and aggression, and cultural patterning of sex-role behavior. She notes in particular the belief in "self-sacrifice" by wives and mothers that women internalize as an ideal difficult to actualize. Canino (1982), in a paper written before she obtained the results of her psychiatric epidemiological (DIS) study, suggests that both men and women have distressful experiences related to sexual dysfunction, and women experience even more distress associated with postpartum experiences and menopause.

When we examine the prevalence of anxiety disorders, as reported by Canino and her colleagues (1987a), we find that women have significantly higher lifetime and six-month rates for phobic disorders, particularly in the subcategories of simple phobia ("persistent fear of a circumscribed stimulus [object or situation] other than fear of having a panic attack or of humiliation" [APA, 1987:243]) and agoraphobia ("fear of being in places or situations from which escape might be difficult" [APA, 1987:241]). However, men and women have about the same rates for panic and obsessive-compulsive disorders. As will be described in Chapter 9 through the use of case material on women with anxiety disorders, women's negative sense of self, augmented by restrictive social mores and situations devolving upon women, in part explains the gender effect on the rates of phobias.

It is of considerable interest that symptoms of panic disorder as defined by DSMIIIR (shortness of breath, dizziness, heart palpitations, trembling, sweating, choking, nausea or abdominal distress, depersonalization, numbness or tingling sensations, flushes or chills, chest pain, fears of dying or going crazy [APA, 1987]) overlap with a popular syndrome labeled as "nervousness." Guarnaccia and his colleagues (1989b) suggest parallels between the popular complaint of *ataque de nervios* (attack of nerves) and the diagnostic category of panic disorder. Both psychiatric and popular ways of categorizing and labeling distress can be said to define the experiences of suffering men and women.

Schizophrenic Disorders

The results of the Diagnostic Interview Schedule study carried out by Canino and colleagues (1987a) show that schizophrenic disorders have a lifetime prevalence rate of 1.8 percent and a six-month prevalence rate of 1.7 percent for women. Rates of schizophrenia in men are somewhat higher than those in women (2.2 percent and 1.4 percent, respectively). People with less than twelve years of education also have somewhat higher rates.

An early study by Rogler and Hollingshead (1965) explored the relationship between family roles and schizophrenia. It examined factors in family life that could cause the disorder, described the impact on the family of a schizophrenic spouse, and explored the effects of family relationships and situations on the chronic course of the illness. Sample families included those with one or two schizophrenic parents and were matched with families without a mentally ill member. All people studied were from the lowest socioeconomic stratum in Puerto Rico; their circumstances were comparable to those of some of the people whose cases are reported in the present study, although a few upper-lower-class and middle-class people were also included. After providing a wealth of descriptive detail vividly describing the lives of these slum families, Rogler and Hollingshead conclude that there are almost no significant differences in the circumstances or interpersonal dynamics of the natal families of mentally ill people and those who raised children who did not become schizophrenic. All of the slum families (with and without schizophrenic members) suffered numerous difficulties associated with poverty.

Although these authors found few differences in the life histories of schizophrenic men and women as compared with nonschizophrenic people, one significant difference was that the former group experienced more frequent nightmares in childhood. Apart from this finding, it seems that all the people they interviewed suffered the same life crises, different in content for men and women, as would be expected given rather sharp differentiation in sex roles. An important finding of the Rogler study is that mentally ill people suffered a problematic year of many crises just prior to the onset of their illness. This resulted in their being unable to carry out work roles, which in turn brought on a pervasive sense of personal inadequacy.

Somatoform Disorders, the Body, and Sexuality

Research concerning experiences of the body and sexuality in Puerto Rico is rather rare. The epidemiological literature shows how readily distress is communicated through bodily references. (See Garrison, 1977a; Srole et al., 1962; Dohrenwend, 1967). Canino's (1988) report, based on the DIS study in Puerto Rico, shows that men and women present almost equal numbers of somatic symptoms. The overall number of such symptoms is significantly higher than among Mexican-Americans in California and also significantly higher than in other ECA populations (whites and blacks) in the United States. When controlled for level of education, equality between men and women in numbers of somatic symptoms and rates of somatization disorder is lost (lifetime prevalence rates are 0.7 percent for both men and women), given the higher educational status of women in Puerto Rico. Age is another important variable. Mean numbers of somatic symptoms are highest (3.5) in women over forty years of age, second highest in men over forty years of age (mean number is 2.3), third highest in women under forty years of age (mean number is 2.1), and lowest in men under 40 years of age (mean number is 1.7). There are no significant differences in the expression of somatic symptoms between younger, less-educated men and women, but there is a definite trend toward older men reporting fewer somatic symptoms as compared with older women. Rates of somatization disorder are significantly lower for groups studied with the same instrument (Diagnostic Interview Schedule) in the United States; perhaps both men and women in Puerto Rico have "amplifying somatizing styles" for expressing malaise rather than many symptoms indicative of disease (Barsky and Klerman, 1983). Being older seems to bring out more somatic complaints.

The DIS study gives a prevalence rate of 26.3 percent for psychosexual dysfunction in Puerto Rico, using the standard version of measurement used in the U.S. studies. Lifetime prevalence rates are 15.9 percent for men and 35.6 percent for women. Because of such high rates, Canino and her colleagues (1987b; Bravo et al., 1991) thought it necessary to modify the algorithm and added questions to the original instrument for the purpose of assessing whether reported "lack of sexual desire" is a criterion that can be scored as indicating disorder. Respondents were asked if the condition of "lack of sexual desire" caused distress to self or partner. The revised criteria lowered the rate of psychosexual disorder to 5.0 percent, a more "reasonable" prevalence figure. The original rates and the dramatic changes in rates can perhaps be explained as due (at least in part) to salient differences between most men and women: men are much more interested and involved with their sexuality to the exclusion of concern about their partners' satisfaction, and many women are ambivalent (and often distressed) about most aspects of sexual behavior, especially in the context of marriage.

Naturally Occurring Complaints of Women: Complaint Profiles

Here I present data on the most frequent complaints of the large opportunity sample of 990 cases seen in treatment by participants in the Therapist-Spiritist Project. These complaints are analysed as key elements of symbolic domains common to discourse about particular categories of psychiatric illness or types of distress, encoded in interactions concerning illness and distress, as recorded in the various health and mental health clinics and Spiritist healing centers.

Methodological Approach

The general approach to this analysis of patients' complaints is that of semantic network analysis following Good and Good (1982:148), who define it as "based on an understanding of meaning as configurations or semantic fields which link key public symbols both to primary social values and to personal affects." Complaint profiles for the four psychiatric higher-rank categories, the deferred diagnosis category, and a nonpsychiatric (medical) category were generated in a multivariate discriminant analysis of 770 cases of women seen by mental health care providers, psychiatrists, and medical doctors (see Appendix, Table A.1, which describes the profiles). There are statistically significant differences between complaint profiles that typify each of the seven categories (see Appendix, "Methodology" and Table A.2).[2]

The profiles generated by the analysis are composed of core complaints that are at the center of a complex made up of a number of personal and social meanings, stressful life events, interpersonal problems, distress in specific parts of the body, failures in social role expectations, or moral dilemmas. (See Good et al., 1985.) Each complex differs according to variations in a complaint profile typical of one type of experience of distress and a corresponding psychiatric or physical category of illness. For example, in the descriptions of the key symbolic domains in 108 cases of anxiety disorder, frequent life events and stressful situations are discussed, such as loss of a loved one through death or desertion and marital dissolution.

The cases of Spiritist healers' clients were also classified by discriminant function analysis as directly parallel to those with psychiatric diagnoses (see Appendix, Table A.3). I also describe the somewhat different symbolic complexes of Spiritists' clients, based on their most frequent and distinctive complaints.

In this study I use data on patients' and clients' complaints (*quejas*) as a window onto their experience of distress and as a point of departure for examining individual and social meanings and interpretations about these disorders. As pointed out by Kleinman and Good (1985), it is the study of emotional disorders, especially their "sociosomatic" aspects, that illustrates how people are both connected and affected by social conditions and cultural traditions. The use of a large number of cases to classify across healer samples, starting with a psychiatric paradigm in order to develop parallels with Spiritist cases, makes it possible to sort out key components to illuminate and compare the qualitative case descriptions.

I use the quantitative analysis for both therapist and Spiritist cases as an initial road map through what is a morass of details. The Spiritist cases are most complex in that they are typified by metaphoric material involving spirits. Because modern medicine and Spiritism have always interfaced, and psychiatry and Spiritism had just begun to relate informally when the Therapist-Spiritist Project entered on the scene to encourage a more formalized relationship, this method illustrates their natural divisions of labor regarding women who suffer severe distress.

It should be noted here that in contrast to patients bringing their complaints to mental health workers or medical doctors, at a Spiritist *centro* spirits report clients' complaints through mediums. Only then are clients asked to verify whether the spirits' descriptions of their distress actually match their experiences. The mediums may then make more detailed probes. Thus there is clearly a selective process in all treatment settings, guided by the working concepts and practices of particular therapists, doctors, or Spiritist healers, with regard to how patient or client complaints are classified and labeled. Therefore, despite the use of imported diagnostic or etiological concepts, whether psychiatric or Spiritist (both originated in other cultures), the expression and experience of distress takes on a special shape that is influenced by popular notions and traditions about illness, emotions, and healing in Puerto Rico. It is also clear that diagnostic conventions and treatment practices are patterned both by individual healers' styles and by a cultural screen of concepts regarding emotions and problematic behavior. (Compare Kleinman, 1980.)

The rationale for the rather arduous task of fitting these data on individual complaints into patterns limited enough to be interpreted in a quantitative way is that it preserves their original form far better than data collected by administering a standardized symptom checklist. I am aware that my method may well overlook some complaints that might be elicited by a standardized questionnaire. However, in this study I decided to sacrifice comprehensiveness in favor of attempting to quantify natural elements of discourse about the experience of distress. Once having arrived at an understanding of central patterns of discourse (expressions) about particular emotional disorders and distress, the next step could be the construction of a culturally adapted complaint checklist to carry out further analyses of how Puerto Rican culture patterns psychiatric disorder and other types of illness.

Depression

The most frequent complaints encountered in eleven women diagnosed as suffering major depression and one hundred thirty-one diagnosed as suffering dysthymic disorder were, in decreasing order, sleep disturbances, crying jags, headaches, intranquility, nervousness, and hallucinations. Hallucinations are much more common in people with major depressive episodes than in those with dysthymic disorders. Crying jags and headaches are found with almost the same frequency in both disorders. Women diagnosed as dysthymic mention problems with memory and low self-esteem as frequently as hallucinations. They also say—though less frequently—that they have chest or heart problems, think about suicide, are sad, and have too much or too little appetite. Like people suffering from major depression, they, too, "feel depressed" and are often in a "bad mood" (see Table A.1).

The most frequent complaints in depressive illness also occur frequently in the other psychiatric diagnostic categories described in this book, although in different proportions and order of frequency. Each psychiatric category additionally includes some frequent and many less frequent complaints that differ from those of other categories. This results in significantly different patterns of complaints for different types of psychiatric disorder (Table A.1). These patterns are also different for men and women who are diagnosed as suffering from the same psychiatric disorders (see Table A.2).

In the paragraphs that follow I examine each of three core complaints of depressed women (sleep disturbances, headaches, and hallucinations) and two combined complaints (intranquility and nervousness) as hubs of symbolic domains that describe common experiences of dysphoria. In most cases, this syndrome of experiences has been diagnosed in mental health clinics as either "major depression" or "dysphoric disorder" but also characterizes those cases seen by the Spiritist healers that would be diagnosed in a similar manner.[3]

Intranquility and Nervousness

"Intranquility" and "nerves" are the most common expressions grouped under the categories of distress and mental illness; together they make up 83 percent of all complaints in cases of major depression, 63 percent of complaints in women diagnosed by therapists as having "dysthymic disorder," and 64 percent of all complaints in the reclassified Spiritist cases (Table A.3). Reference to nerves or nervousness is by far the most common single complaint, a way of describing experiences of distress that include a somatic referent. To be nervous implies that one's total being is "disturbed," "shook up," "out of control," "lacking serenity or peace." There are various grades of severity and some variations in the general condition of "nervousness"; most women say they feel "*bien nerviosa*" (very nervous), which commonly indicates severe distress, although this is not as serious as suffering from "having nerves" or being "sick from nerves." These expressions can be oblique references to "craziness" or psychosis or indicate an anxiety disorder. A guide to how this type of distress feels is indicated by other, closely related expressions of complaint: intranquility (*inquietud*), anxiety (*ansiedad*), worry or disquiet (*desasociego*), and agitation (*agitación*).

Some of these expressions are similar to complaints also reported as frequent in depressive disorders in women in the continental United States—particularly irritability and decreased ability to concentrate. However, the meanings associated with the "nerves-intranquility" complex do not include other equally common symptoms of depression of women in the United States, such as social withdrawal and lowered levels of activity ("vegetative signs"). They point instead to a prominent "agitated" dimension to dysphoric mood.[4]

Sleep Disturbances and Hallucinations

Sleep disturbances and hallucinations account for almost half of all complaints in therapist cases diagnosed as major depression, three-fourths of complaints in therapist cases diagnosed as dysthymic disorder, and only approximately one-fourth of complaints in parallel Spiritist cases, where "hallucinations" as a complaint doesn't appear at all.[5] Sleep disturbances are a very common complaint across diagnostic categories. Particular complaints are "insomnia" or "sleepiness" (hypersomnia) but even more frequently "nightmares" expressed as "lying" dreams, "strange" dreams, and occasionally as "sleepwalking." The reason for combining these two complaints within one symbolic domain is that they are both linked to fears about one's death or the death of one's children.

*Crying Jags (*Ataques de Llanto*)*

Frequent and prolonged crying appears to be a common complaint in cases falling into all of the psychiatric categories, except that of personality disorders. But it occurs most frequently in both therapist and Spiritist cases of dysthymic disorder and somewhat less frequently in cases of major depression. Crying due to grief over loss (especially through death or abandonment) is expected behavior in Puerto Rico, and much sympathy goes out to the sufferer. Apart from this kind of event, crying is not well tolerated; it seems to arouse much more discomfort than sympathy.

Headaches

Headaches (including pain and pulsations at the back of the head, "migraine," stabbing pains in the head, feelings that the head will burst, sensations that the head is swollen, or needles or stabbing pains in the forehead or head) are the third most frequent complaint in psychiatric categories of depression among women being seen by therapists and Spiritists. (Headaches head the list of complaints in nonpsychiatric cases.) Headaches are found approximately equally in people diagnosed as suffering major depression and in people with dysthymic disorder. They are somewhat more frequent in Spiritist cases reclassified as dysthymic disorder. Regardless of possible cause, which may vary from physical to psychogenic, "headache" is the key symbol in a domain that describes how emotional distress occurs. "Headache" frequently refers to distress caused by the moods, thoughts, or actions of other people, particularly those with whom one is in conflict.

Complaints Specific to Spiritist Clients with Depression

Chest and heart pains are a small percentage of the dysthymic disorders complaint profile in therapist cases. In contrast, in Spiritist patients backaches and leg aches are fairly frequent. Spiritist healers regularly talk about and attend to body complaints associated with dysphoric mood or other types of emotional disturbance. The most frequent reasons healers "see" for a spirit invading a woman who would be diagnosed as depressed are as follows: The spirit wants to cause an illness or operation; it wishes to harm the client; it has a vengeance motive because of past life events; it wants to isolate the client, break up her marriage, or cause death.

Feeling "fearful" and crying jags are the two most frequent complaints in Spiritist cases of depression. They imply that a large component of the discourse on dysphoric affect in Spiritist clients is fear about physical survival—fear of serious illness or even death—as will be described in Chapter 7.

Schizophrenia

In the sample of 488 cases of women in treatment in mental health clinics, about 15 percent were diagnosed as suffering a schizophrenic disorder. Their median age was twenty-nine years. (See Appendix, Tables A.1, A.2, A.3, and A.4.) Their most frequent complaints were, in decreasing order, sleep disturbances, hallucinations, hostility, intranquility, head pains, nervousness, crying jags, and feelings of depression. In contrast, there was only one Spiritist case in the sample of 220 cases that could be reclassified as "schizophrenia," and this included the common complaint of "marital and family problems." "Hostility" is the only complaint that distinguishes the list of complaints of people with schizophrenia from that of people with major depression; hallucinations and sleep disturbances appeared with approximately the same frequency in both groups. Because certain types of hallucinations and delusions are important to confirming a diagnosis of psychosis in mental health clinics, in a culture such as Puerto Rico where visions are perceived as unusual but "normal," expectable experiences, there appears at times to be some confusion about identifying hallucinations—even among psychiatric diagnosticians. As is already evident to the reader, visions and other nonordinary experiences are positive for Spiritist healers and also of central importance in promoting personal transformation.

"Hostility" and "hallucinations/delusions," as complaints, are key symbols in semantic and behavioral complexes that typify the experience of schizophrenia in women in Puerto Rico. "Hostility" (including anger) was found in almost half of the women diagnosed as having a schizophrenic disorder among the women in treatment in mental health clinics. Hostile feelings and behavior in women seem to be particularly associated with failures in mother-daughter relationships. Perceived rejection by a daughter, coupled with domination of the young woman by her mother, is a common situation, even among normal people. A mother's fears about a daughter's sexual license and early loss of virginity (which bring shame to the family) sometimes lead to exaggerated attempts to restrict the daughter's freedom, which can produce intense conflict. I am not implying that such failures in relationship between mothers and daughters cause mental disorder, only that they are often associated with expressions of hostility in women and surface as a complaint once a daughter is severely emotionally disturbed. Schizophrenic women, once ill, also express hostility toward their own daughters, whom they perceive as rejecting and abandoning.

Hallucinations and delusions are not exclusively symptoms of schizophrenia but also occur in 15 percent of people suffering manic-depressive illness. "Delusions" are defined in the Diagnostic and Statistical Manual (DSMIIIR, APA, 1987) as having "content patently absurd" with "no possible basis in fact." "Hallucinations" are defined as major disturbances in perception, of which the auditory variety are the most common in schizophrenics. Somatic and visual hallucinations are much less frequent but not rare. In the cases of women diagnosed in our sample as having a schizophrenic disorder, a few less than one-half presented with hallucinations or delusions. Hallucinations are absent from the one Spiritist case classified as schizophrenia by the computer analysis, which is the main reason why so few Spiritist cases could be reclassified as "schizophrenia."

Anxiety Disorders

In the sample of 770 cases of women seen by both medical doctors and mental health therapists, "anxiety disorder" was the most frequent psychiatric diagnosis. There were 108 people so diagnosed, six by medical doctors. As

UNIV DUNELM

will be noted by those familiar with the American Psychiatric Association's diagnostic manuals, "panic disorder" does not appear in the 1968 version (DSMII, APA); but it was commonly diagnosed in Puerto Rico as "anxiety reaction with hysterical features" or was included under general "anxiety reaction." "Obsessive-compulsive disorder" was often diagnosed as a "personality disorder," and "phobia" does not appear in the earlier diagnostic classifications. However, descriptions of symptoms collected from patients or presented to the case discussion sessions of the Therapist-Spiritist Project certainly point to phobic behavior. Given the morass of changes in diagnostic fashions, I have chosen to lump all therapists' diagnoses into one higher-rank category, "anxiety disorders," that subsumes variations in separately defined subcategories, such as specific phobias. Variations will be mentioned in relation to individual cases only when they seem significant.

Among the reclassified Spiritist women's cases, there were fifty-one with the complaint profile of the "anxiety disorders" category, an even higher percentage than among cases seen by mental health workers. Although they show considerable overlap, the complaint profiles of therapist and Spiritist cases differ in interesting ways.

"Sleep disturbances" appear in about half of the cases (insomnia, sleepwalking, nightmares, "strange" and "lying" dreams, and sleep disturbances in general). They head the list as the most frequent type of complaint of therapist patients. They are much less frequent in Spiritist clients (appearing in less than one-fifth of the cases). In contrast, "mind" problems (for example, mind is "blank," "dark," "molested," "in turmoil," "gone," "tired," "disturbed," "overloaded," "running on," "bewildered," or "stalled") head the complaint list for just under one-half of the Spiritist clients in the anxiety disorder category. Individual complaints of "nervousness," "intranquility" and "head problems/headaches" are presented as frequently by therapist patients as by Spiritist clients. However, therapist patients also commonly present with somewhat frequent "crying jags," "hostility/anger/aggressiveness," "hallucinations," and "trembling." Instead of these complaints, Spiritist clients commonly present with "fatigue," "chest/heart problems," and "family problems." This last complaint is associated with the very different approach of the Spiritist healers toward physical and mental illness; they usually focus equally on a client's social (external) and personal (internal) difficulties. In addition, clients at *centros* are more focused on their bodies (including "minds") as sites in which they experience disorder and malaise, as compared with mental health clients.

Although intranquility and nervousness are a large part of discourse and experience in relation to depression, the particular ways "intranquility" and "nerves" appear in the presentations of women with anxiety disorders are somewhat different, as will be described in Chapter 9.

"Headache" (including the many kinds of head pain listed previously) is the second most frequent complaint of women diagnosed as suffering from anxiety disorders. People with severe headaches, sometimes accompanied by heart palpitations, commonly present first to medical doctors before they seek other help. "Headaches" and other somatic symptoms are often associated with family and work problems, and the sufferer feels trapped by a situation in which she perceives that losing her job threatens her very survival.

Approximately one-fourth of the women who come to Spiritist sessions, whose complaint profiles paralleled those of mental health clients diagnosed with anxiety disorders, presented with "fatigue" (including various forms of bodily weakness) and "chest/heart pains." These complaints may accompany panic disorder as part of a syndrome of extreme motor tension and autonomic hyperactivity. Canino and her colleagues (1987b) list chest pain as the second of the five most common panic symptoms, which also include palpitations, fear of dying or going crazy, choking, and sweating.

Somatoform Disorders

As expected from the results of the epidemiological studies, somatoform disorders were not frequent in our sample of cases. There were thirteen therapist cases and sixteen reclassified Spiritist cases classified by computer analysis as somatoform disorders. These types of cases are not easily diagnosed because of their resemblance to depression, especially major depression where diffuse somatic complaints are thought by psychiatrists to substitute for the expression of dysphoric affect (Katon et al., 1982).

Frequent complaints in this profile are "nervousness" and "intranquility." These complaints have mixed somatic and physical referents and seem to distinguish patients and clients who are psychologically impaired and who use physical complaints to express disordered feelings and emotions from those with minor physical illnesses (many also with psychological aspects). However, separating out persons suffering psychological impairment expressed as preoccupation with the body is extremely difficult given Puerto Ricans' pattern of expressing much of their malaise in somatic terms. Note also that doctors in most medical clinics rarely asked about or recorded psychosocial distress (which we observed in their case report write-ups).

Deferred Psychiatric Diagnosis

Approximately one-eighth of the mental health patients and a similar fraction of the reclassified Spiritist clients presented for help with emotional distress but were not diagnosed (or diagnosable) as having a psychiatric illness. In this category, the complaint profile of mental health patients is headed by sleep disturbances, headaches, crying jags, and nervousness; this profile is very similar to the depression profiles. However, two unique complaints—

"fright" and "eye/vision problems"—appear in about 10 percent of the cases of mental health clinic patients. This is the only profile in which these two complaints are frequent.[6]

It seems that therapist cases in the "deferred diagnosis" category are mainly instances of mental health clinicians being confused about diagnosing and treating particular patients. In addition, doctors reported that they sometimes found these patients to have "irritating" personal characteristics, such as "belief in spirits," chronic complaining naming many different body parts, or complicating interpersonal problems. Spiritists also "deferred" (and referred to medical doctors) when they could not cope with a severely mentally ill person. In contrast, mental health professionals expressed doubts about intervening with clients who did not appear to be severely impaired, usually because of lack of time.

No Psychiatric Diagnosis

There were 403 mental health and medical cases and 104 reclassified Spiritist cases grouped by the analysis into the "no-psychiatric diagnosis" category. The complaint profile for these cases with mainly physical complaints contains the longest list of most frequent somatic symptoms. (See Appendix, Table A.1 for a list of complaints and their frequencies.) Somatic complaints for this category include headaches as do all the other profiles, but also stomach problems, fever, throat problems, dizzy spells, chest/heart problems, leg/feet problems, fatigue, hypertension, back problems, and change in appetite—in descending order of frequency. The list also includes intranquility and hostility, as well as many other mood complaints, but in low frequencies.

There are fewer types of somatic complaints in the profile of the "no psychiatric diagnosis" category for Spiritist cases. Instead marital and family problems are frequent complaints. Spiritists tend to "read" body symptoms as metaphors for interpersonal distress if they diagnose the problem as spiritually caused. However, the total number of somatic complaints in individual cases (and complaints in general) presented to (more accurately, "captured by") Spiritists is frequently large. Some Spiritist clients present as many as twenty-two to twenty-eight bodily complaints.

We can only speculate about which cases in the "no psychiatric diagnosis" category (including medical cases) are organic in etiology and presentation and which are examples of what medicine calls "psychosomatic" illness. The 5 percent that present with "hostility" and the 6 percent that present with "intranquility" may indicate that 11 percent of medical patients have what has been called "functional somatic symptoms," that is, psychological reactions to stress expressed through the body. Spiritists make no such distinction, because by tradition and belief they are unconcerned with "psychological" causality of bodily or other symptoms. Instead they view most distress as spirit caused rather than mediated by the mind/psyche. They do not assume that somatic complaints are displacements of negative emotions from interior states to overt, verbal signs of distress. Of the Spiritist cases in this study, close to three-fourths were diagnosed as having either "spiritual causes" or a mixture of material and spiritual causes.

Summary

The preceding descriptions of types of mental illness and emotional disorder in Puerto Rico are aimed at setting the stage for recalling the experiences of women as patients and clients. These experiences are presented in the next four chapters. In those chapters I have grouped together women in mental health care, medical treatment, and Spiritist treatment. My reason for doing so is that these women share an overall pattern of distressful experience typified by expressions of feeling and notions that describe their common experience as women. However, there are differences in the frequency, emphasis, and response to complaints that tell us about variations on patterns of distress and suffering that are largely held in common. The discriminant analysis of the complaint profiles shows that somewhat more than half of the women who present to the Spiritists (104 out of 220 cases) would either fall within the group of patients that mental health workers do not diagnose (or chose to defer diagnosing) or have complaints similar to those who present to public health or family medicine clinics. These cases are described in Chapter 10 where attitudes and distress expressed in bodily terms, including those severe enough to be classified in psychiatric manuals as somatoform disorders, are discussed.

Somewhat more than half of the problems Spiritists see (116 out of 220 cases) are diagnosable as psychiatric disorders in the higher-rank categories I have examined. (The reader will note that I have not explored the cases categorized as "personality disorders" because of the complexities within this category.) One might appreciate that most of these cases are similar to, although many are not as severe as, some of the psychiatrically diagnosed cases. However, there are many complexities to the system of seeking help for emotional and behavioral problems, which will be described in the next four chapters. The analysis of case material based on psychiatric categories as a starting point makes it possible to appreciate the work of the Spiritists as partly overlapping that of the mental health professionals and also that of the medical doctors. More important, the work of the Spiritists is also partly distinct, because Spiritist healers regularly deal with the less severe emotional and physical complaints ("deferred" and "no diagnosis" categories) that mental health professionals and medical doctors often do not treat. Thus Spiritist healing practices take up the slack left by the community mental health system, which defines its principal mandate as serving persons suffering from psychiatric illness.

A major aim of the presentations that follow is to provide the reader with a close view of how varying explanations of emotional and behavioral distress, held by different types of healers, have implications for all aspects of treatment, such as defining the distress, the content and direction of the discourse among all parties to the treatment (including families and friends), the prognosis, the outcome, and, perhaps most important, how the distress and its resolution is experienced by the sufferer. In addition, the exploration of contrasting interpretations of similar moods, feelings, and behavior by mental health professionals, medical doctors, and Spiritist healers provides a way to understand how Puerto Rican culture transforms certain basic human experiences of pain, disorientation, and despair through both noncognitive and symbolic modes. As Kleinman and Kleinman so eloquently express in their study of the cultural patterning of depression in China, these comparisons illuminate "the sociosomatic reticulum (the symbolic bridge) that connects individuals to each other and their life world" (1985:429). I might add that they also illustrate disconnections from that world even more clearly.

My focus in Chapters 7 through 10 is on how women as patients and clients experience and express emotional and physical malaise with all of their complexities, variations, and, at times, vagaries. I also attempt an understanding of how their malaise is rooted in the difficulties that inhere in women's roles in Puerto Rico, resonating not only with values, assumptions, economic conditions, and gender expectations but also with ambivalences and ambiguities about women. This book uses help seeking and a clinical lens as one route to understanding gender-related problems.

The four strands of interpretation described in Chapter 1 are used in describing the experiences of patients and clients of the healers. The first strand is that of the healers talking about themselves in relation to their work with patients and clients; the second is that of healers' accounts of their patients and clients; the third is that of patients and clients talking about their own experiences of distress and illness, including their experiences of treatment and healing; and the fourth is composed of the interpretations of Project events made by Hector and me, as well as our comments, based on published studies, that amplify the first three strands of interpretation.

Notes

1. The Diagnostic Interview Schedule (DIS) is based upon DSMIII (APA, 1980). It measures only those psychiatric disorders with highest expected prevalence in a population. It focuses principally on higher-rank (general) categories of psychiatric disorder. Bravo et al., 1991, discuss the ways Canino and her colleagues adapted the instrument to Puerto Rico.

2. My method used six general, psychiatric categories (major depression, dysthymia, schizophrenia, somatoform and dissociative disorders, anxiety disorders, and personality disorders) as well as two residual categories (no psychiatric diagnosis and deferred diagnosis) (see Appendix, Table A.1). Although DSMII diagnoses (APA, 1968) were used by the mental health workers studied in 1976–1979, the four higher-rank categories I examine group specific psychiatric diagnoses to reflect changes in the newer DSMIIIR (APA, 1987) diagnostic divisions. Multivariate tests show significant main effects between gender and diagnostic categories as well as significant interactions between these variables (see Table A.2). In other words, males and females in Puerto Rico present different complaint profiles over all psychiatric and nonpsychiatric categories. It must be noted that these naturally occurring complaint profiles are not the same as symptom lists or behavioral disturbances described in psychiatric diagnostic manuals such as DSMIIIR as criteria with which to make a diagnosis, although they do overlap with these criteria. Both parallels and differences are noted in following chapters.

The data collected for the present study are not based on probability samples and therefore cannot be used to compare rates found in the DIS/ECA studies. It is of interest, however, that the incidence of affective and anxiety disorders (which included cases of psychosexual dysfunction and phobia) show similar trends. In the DIS study in Puerto Rico, the number of male cases of major depression is only slightly smaller than the number of female cases, but female cases of dysthymia are 4.75 times those of males. In the very different type of study presented in this book (clinical as compared with a random community sample), cases of dysthymic disorder in women number somewhat more than twice those of men in the 1,769 cases in the entire sample of males and females used for the quantitative analysis (see Appendix, Table A.2). Because there were too few cases of alcohol abuse or dependence and cognitive impairment in the data we collected, an exploration of these disorders is not included in this book. A specific finding of the DIS study is that women have much lower rates of alcoholism and drug abuse than men in Puerto Rico and somewhat lower rates than at other ECA sites, where women also have fewer problems of substance abuse. In addition, although I constructed complaint profiles for the category "personality disorder," I do not describe the central features or experiences of women so diagnosed because the category has a number of important subdivisions (antisocial personality disorder, paranoid personality disorder, and so on), and I did not have enough case material (particularly for Spiritist clients) to explore these complexities.

3. Although these particular complaints predominate in discourse about depressive disorders between patients and mental health professionals in Puerto Rico, they are not generally considered in psychiatric nosology to be core systems of affective disorders. Similar core complaints do appear in psychiatrically diagnosed and other people in other cultural settings (see Kleinman and Good, 1985), but the ways core and less-frequent complaints articulate with notions, attitudes, life situations, and linked feelings to form a network or complex around a pattern of experience appears to be unique to Puerto Rican women. This is expected because differences in expressions about dysphoric feelings depend upon the meanings particular complaints and associated experiences have for these women. In turn, the expression of these manifestations of distress, that is, a profile of sleep disturbances, headaches, intranquility, nervousness, and hallucinations of *celajes* (ghosts), determines how the women

or their relatives interpret and assess feelings of distress judged severe enough to require help from a mental health professional or a nonmedical healer.

4. It can be noted that a large number of cases in the quantitatively analyzed sample of 990 cases of women who sought help for emotional complaints were diagnosed as "neurotic depression with features of anxiety" or "depressive anxiety reaction" (DSMII, APA, 1968). Lehmann points out that "virtually all depressed patients suffer from anxiety," the "two states exist together" (1985:793). My data suggest that they are inextricably intertwined in depressive states in Puerto Rico, particularly among women. The cultural ambience fosters both intense sociality and extensive social networks that potentially protect against social isolation and feelings of alienation. On the other hand, this same pattern of social relationships almost inevitably fosters anxiety, because the depressed actress must constantly mask her desire not to be socially responsive.

5. As will be discussed in subsequent chapters, "to hallucinate" is not a concept that has meaning for Spiritist believers, who interpret "nonreal," nonpresent phenomena as visions of spirits that may or may not connote illness or emotional distress.

6. Garrison (1977a), using the Cornell Medical Index to look at complaints that the people in her New York Puerto Rican sample took to a doctor, reports that 55 percent found no help with eye problems. This was the most frequent type of complaint leading to dissatisfaction with medical care; urogenital complaints ran a close second. Garrison also describes the commonness of gynecological concerns in her sample of fifty Spiritist clients. Later I argue that these kinds of complaints are focal points of much of the bodily distress expressed by women.

7

Dysphoric Mood and Depression

Women's second-class position in patriarchal culture is painfully reflected in their psychology. Women do not feel whole; women do not feel confident in themselves; women feel less than equal; women feel like children, not adults; women feel powerless; women feel overdependent; women feel passive; women feel imprisoned by their anger and by the clouds of depression that often surround them.

—L. Eichenbaum and S. Orbach, *Understanding Women*

An outsider observing groups of people at the airport, at restaurants, or at special places where students congregate near a university in Puerto Rico will be struck by the atmosphere of gaiety, excitement, and goodwill that seems to typify group life in public places. At informal social gatherings or in encounters between friends in the course of the day, everyone appears to be cheery, relaxed, full of smiles and even laughter. It is not uncommon to walk down a busy city street and hear fellow pedestrians singing or catch the banter of friendly joking issuing from an open patio. A high priority is placed on projecting happiness and well-being when presenting oneself to people outside one's most intimate circle.

The social requirement of euphoric response is imposed early in a child's life, as epitomized in the encounter of a woman and an infant who has not yet begun to produce the desired facial expressions. The woman will almost invariably squeeze the infant's cheeks in order to elicit a smile. Optimism, hopefulness, and at least outward exuberance are clearly favored responses to the much-talked-about difficulties associated with living in Puerto Rico—the much-feared crime, a high cost of living, an uncertain economy, frequent automobile accidents, and far-reaching, rapid social and cultural changes, among other problems. The depth of this popular attitude toward a euphoric response to life's difficulties can be appreciated in the lyrics of a song that is still a national favorite, "El Jibarito." This is a pre-World War II lament (at times almost tearful) of a poor country farmer who goes to market in an exuberant mood. Later, finding that he cannot sell his goods, he returns home crying that his wife and children will not have the small gifts he so joyously had promised—and will probably starve. But, as expected, the song ends on the optimistic note that he *knows* all will be well in time.

Given the preferred ethos of euphoria that dominates public expression in Puerto Rico, most people tend to use a "pleasing" style of response to everyday events and expect in turn to receive positive emotional expressions in most social situations. On the other side of this proverbial coin, the definition of desirable behavior also includes a strong injunction against the expression of anger and a desire to avoid any situation involving conflict. But these ideals are submerged in almost infinite difficulties and contradictions. For example, almost everyone thinks of himself or herself as an independent, free "individual," yet tradition supports a high degree of conformity, as if Puerto Rican society was still a small, highly integrated community. While small communities were more the rule than the exception some decades ago, very few still exist in the densely populated, tightly urbanized island of the nineties. Angry, aggressive behavior is still strongly disapproved within intimate or extended family circles and continues to be suppressed in some communities, thus following the social guidelines characteristic of a traditional, sociocentric culture.

The paradox for Puerto Ricans is that preindustrial community life has practically disappeared, and individual families more or less have to survive by their own efforts. Most people attempt to preserve the supportive, interdependent structure of the traditional extended family, finding it to be a more and more difficult undertaking. As always, the positive image of "community" or of "extended family" mutuality seems to live on, even though its patent ephemerality is encountered more and more. (For example, it is a fairly common expectation that siblings or grown children will migrate to the continental United States.) As a result, there are now very few effective family or community controls over violent or deviant behavior occasioned by drinking, delinquency, or mental illness.

The Expression of Dysphoria

Disapproval of assertive behavior or expressions of anger in women is practically societywide. Almost any public demonstration of agressiveness shames the family. Gossip, often malicious (*bochinches*), seems to substitute for overt angry feelings, especially among women as neighbors or coworkers.[1] In direct contrast, it is *expected* that men will have intensely angry outbursts whenever a stressful incident causes them to exceed their limits for storage of anger; fist fights and sometimes even the brandishing (and shooting) of weapons occur in traffic jams. A central issue for men is the need to control their emotions, because they continually threaten to erupt in ways that might undermine other people's opinions of their worth as "good men" and bring on unwanted difficulties. For women, however, angry and aggressive feelings are heavily suppressed from childhood onward, with few outlets (Wolf, 1952; Torres-Matrullo, 1982).

One possible outlet for women, suggested by the large number of somatic complaints elicited by symptom checklists of all kinds, is the opportunity to give vent to repressed feelings of anger and frustration in the form of a "rhetoric of complaint." In Chapter 5 I alluded to an interesting perspective suggested by Gaines and Farmer (1986) (which they generalize to the Caribbean as linked to the Mediterranean culture area), who describe how some lower-class French women acquire reputations as "social cynosures" because they publicly parade a chronic liturgy of suffering. Their martyrdom is positively supported by Catholic images of suffering saints. Gaines interprets this situation as representing the cultural incorporation of a state of dysphoria not considered deviant or abnormal but treated as an accepted feeling of sadness or a "state of fatigue" with life. In Puerto Rico, some middle-aged women also cry about past losses and parade their complaints of illness. However, they are usually met with covert or polite rejection if they do so frequently. These women are nicknamed *lloronas* (crybabies) and jokingly derogated. Rather than evoking sympathy, excessive complaining makes others feel uncomfortable. It *is* acceptable, even applauded, if mothers talk about the sacrifices and difficulties they have experienced in rearing children. But they must always appear to be in the process of winning out over the difficulties associated with that sacred task.

With regard to the public exercise of euphoric mood, although much of it is genuine and socializing is highly enjoyed (certainly engaged in with fervor and frequency), a good deal of it amounts to social form, yet it did not appear to me to be forced or obligatory. It seems likely that widely shared expressions of well-being in a fiesta-like atmosphere are actually therapeutic. Fears and disquiet about the resolution of problems can stay at the back of one's mind, at least for the moment, to be replaced by positive feelings evoked in the generally pleasurable ambience of social intercourse.

Running counter to the positive effects of socializing is a covert agreement that people can affect each other in excessive and negative ways. A number of old beliefs attest to this view, such as the notion that small children can be harmed by persons who consciously or inadvertently turn the evil eye (*mal de ojo*) upon them either through jealousy or too much admiration. Most educated people scoff at such ideas but can be easily urged by the caretakers of their children to buy *azabaches*, charms against evil influence emanating from strangers who lavish special attention upon their children.

Beliefs in witchcraft, described in Chapter 5, are also testimony to culturally constituted feelings about invasive, unwanted affect. The pervasiveness of discomfort caused by another person's perceived envy, anger, or distrust may be the source of the many witchcraft accusations that are difficult to substantiate. As we were often reminded, the central conviction of those who believe in Spiritism, that illness is inflicted upon the sufferer by backward or misguided spirits, is also based on the implicit premise that one's very being is eternally vulnerable to penetration by external, negative influences.

In most of the Spiritist cases—especially in those dealing with serious physical illness—healers interpret complaints as coming from a spirit who suffered the same distress while incarnate. This perspective, that the cause of illness is a human or spirit agent outside the body, is analyzed in the literature on Hispanic peoples as due to an "external locus of control" theory of disease attribution. Mirowsky and Ross (1984), in a study of Mexican Americans in Texas, suggest that belief in an external locus of control in part stems from a sociocentric orientation, that is, where high priority is given to mutual obligations and responsibilities among relatives and friends. This then leads to a sense of limited personal autonomy, loss of personal control, and vulnerability to depression. However, these authors point out that the negative aspects of this type of social orientation are balanced by the way a large social support network functions to lessen anxiety. They imply that loss of social support would increase anxiety but decrease depression. While I agree with Mirowsky's and Ross's general perspective, its validity requires illustration in specific situations of distress and in particular groups. The narratives I present below show how precarious this interpersonal balancing act can be. It seems to work in far more complex ways than Mirowsky's and Ross's general formulation suggests. Moreover, such formulations overlook the psychological significance of a cultural pattern that fosters a high degree of interdependence among nuclear family members, commonly expressed as intense emotional enmeshment.

Canino and Canino (1982), in discussing family therapy for Puerto Rican migrant families, characterize the Puerto Rican family as "normally enmeshed," although it may appear to be abnormally so to North American therapists. Various discussions of the mother-child relationship in Puerto Rico describe its characteristic closeness and continuity, even into adulthood (Nieves Falcon, 1973). Some investigators have interpreted this family pattern as leading to psychopathological reactions in sons of mothers who wish to absorb their male offspring (Fernández Marina et al., 1958; Maldonado Sierra et al., 1960). I suggest that these analyses overlook the "normal" emotional environment created in most Puerto Rican families that encourages a high degree of shared affect and interdependence among its members. I found evidence of few accepted psychological barriers between parents and children. Given this patterning of the family environment, individuals observe their familial responsibilities because they have internalized pressing motives for doing so.

Why then is depression as a psychiatric disorder even more prevalent among women than men in Puerto Rico as compared with its prevalence in U.S. communities (Canino et al., 1987b)? Yet depression is equally prevalent among men in Puerto Rico and the United States. How does the presence of a disorder typified by variations in dysphoric mood relate to the importance placed upon gaiety and happiness, especially in public and extrafamilial social settings? In particular, why do women, as compared with men, suffer almost five times as much dysthymia (defined as a "mood disorder" in DSMIIIR, APA, 1987) over their lifetimes? Does the culturally patterned and enforced habit of suppressing and hoarding dysphoric affect somehow facilitate its later expression in dysfunctional and disordered behavior? Or is the generally positive and expected familial enmeshment (and associated feelings of well-being) offset by lack of social support and by stress-inducing social obligations difficult to meet under postindustrial societal conditions? What precisely is the etiology of the high rates of depression in women?

Experiences of Depression and Dysthymia

My approach to depression among Puerto Rican women is an exploration of the relationships between feelings of distress, feelings of lack of worth as a woman, and problems in sexual and reproductive functioning. In the case descriptions to follow, the reader may observe with me how feelings about reproductive status and motherhood are often central to discourse about distress. Some of these cases were described to us by the patients themselves or by their therapists or Spiritist healers, but most were presented by healer-participants in the case review sessions. The case descriptions elicited sometimes copious comments from other healers of all three types. Again, I ask the reader to be with us at these sessions, to listen and observe as case after case unfolds before us, two in each session and many others during our hundreds of interviews. All of the presenters submitted to the questioning, discussions, conflicting opinions, and practical suggestions of other participants. (The case narratives of presenters were supplemented by interviews.) Clearly only certain highlights can be presented in the next four chapters, but we invite your participation as close observers and your opinions on the interpretations we interject into the narratives of healers about patients and clients and into those of the patients and clients themselves.

Adriana

Adriana's case was presented by Lisa, a mental health technician. She diagnosed her client as suffering "major depression." Lisa recounted:

> Adriana is a thirty-year-old woman, married for seven years to a policeman, with a five-year-old son who was deaf and had speech problems. She said that she was "nervous, had headaches, eye and knee pains, was sad, depressed, didn't

> sleep well, and was afraid of the dark." She also "heard and saw things." Her "family" [a brother and a cousin] "suffered from nerves." Adriana had been hospitalized in the United States for ten days some eight years previously for an *ataque de nervios.* She also suffered a "thrombosis" shortly after she was hospitalized, which she attributes to the pressures of her bosses at her job; she has not worked since that time. Her current [presenting] problems are marital conflict and a quarrel with her father, which has lasted five years—both aggravated by worry over her son's difficulties. She has been seen as an outpatient in the CMHC for five years and is taking antidepressant medication. Adriana's reference to "nerves" is to feeling "nervous," but she acknowledges that the "condition" runs in the family.

We noted that the implication was that Adriana had inherited "nervousness" (as did a sibling and a cousin who, she said, "have nerves") as a chronic disability or defect. Her nervousness could potentially become serious so that she could (and did) completely lose control over her behavior. Hospitalization was the expected consequence. The situation of *nervios* reaching the level of an *ataque* is addressed in more detail in Chapter 9. Here it suffices to note that if a person is thought to have "nerves" as an inborn defect or disability, he or she is believed to be much more vulnerable to dissociative and out-of-control experiences. These are popular notions about the cause and nature of mental disorder that crosscut psychiatric concepts regarding hereditary predispositions.

The healers' comments about Adriana focused on the notion that the experience of "nervousness" is linked to marital conflict, which seems to arouse deep fears of abandonment and inability to survive without a mate. Adriana was said to be a "good example" of how a "nervous" woman can be concerned about her husband's extramarital affairs, especially given the fact that she was his third wife. Lisa responded that she had observed Adriana to feel very insecure, in part related to her inability to work. Other participants suggested that her deep sense of insecurity was the context for her distress about the conflict with her father and that this was further exacerbated by her son's disabilities. (Hector and I noted that the quality of Adriana's fear about personal survival, her almost paranoid preoccupation with death, is central to the symbolic domain of "sleep disturbances" and "hallucinations," as described in the preceding chapter.)

The physical dimension of nervousness as severe distress was well illustrated in a Spiritist healer's *videncia* of one client's distress: She asked this client, "*Tu te sientes en toda la materia, de la cabeza hasta los pies, cómo un nerviosismo?*" (Do you feel a nervousness throughout your entire body from your head to your feet?) The client replied, "Yes, certainly." This client also admitted to feeling "depressed" and "a melancholia." We noted that "nerves" as a reported experience seemed to denote distress that included fears about the very survival of one's physical being.

Claudia

The case of Claudia was presented at a case review session. Her experience of "nerves" seemed directly related to the kinds of fears just discussed. The psychologist-presenter said:

> Claudia is thirty-three years of age, with two children, six and four years old. She has been married for over fifteen years. Her complaints began when she was working as an "operator" in a factory; she said that the pressure of work caused them. She was diagnosed at first as suffering a "schizophrenic reaction with paranoid features," but later this was changed to a diagnosis of "major depression." Claudia lives enclosed within her home and admits to beating her two children because they make her angry. On saying this she cries profusely.
>
> In addition to "nervousness," "fear," "headaches," and "crying jags" (*ataques de llanto*), Claudia's most distressing complaint is that she sees persons who want to kill her children and strangle her. She often sees a man dressed in white, whose feet do not touch the ground. She hears these feared persons murmuring in her ear, is afraid to sleep, and fears the dark. She also sees many eyes that look at her. She takes her children to bed with her and avoids sleeping with her husband. But when she does sleep, she screams a lot because of nightmares. Although afraid to leave the house, she feels a great desire to run away.
>
> Following a two-week course of antidepressive and antipsychotic medications Claudia is no longer experiencing hallucinations, but her other complaints continue.

Participants said they agreed that Claudia's fears prevented her from sleeping because she had to be forever vigilant about her own and her childrens' safety. For her, sleep brought fearful visions of harmful men or disembodied eyes. We noted that in several other severe cases, especially those diagnosed as major depression, sleep disturbances, nightmares, and fears about personal safety were typical. One woman, who complained about insomnia, had the belief (which could not be substantiated and had been labeled as "delusional" by her therapist) that her husband was trying to harm her.[2] These linkages between complaints indicated to us that the experience of sleep disturbance also included severe marital problems and a view of men as threatening or fatally abusive. This view may stem from early experiences with an alcoholic, abusive father. In the experience of Josefa (as she told us), her fearful disposition was associated with a husband who was very abusive and angry with her. One Spiritist healer commented that many women talk about physical abuse at the hands of their husbands and that this directly related to their being "*aguantona*," that is, a person who endures suffering without complaint. We noted that this was a popular notion about femimine personality that is both praised and ambivalently regarded by women themselves.

Josefa

A mental health worker presented the case of Josefa.

> Josefa, fifty-five years of age, has been living with her second mate for fourteen years and has no children. She has a history of depression [current diagnosis, "reactive depression" (DSMII, APA, 1968)], including complaints of feeling depressed, crying a great deal, nightmares, and feelings of great sorrow [*pena*]. She also feels "empty" and has no desire to live. She says that her complaints began some sixteen years ago following a divorce from her first husband, who attempted to strangle her while she slept. She talks about fears of knowing the "reality of her sorrows" and suffering and "becoming crazy." Relations with her present mate are also difficult.

We reflected that linked with excessive crying is a strong sense of emptiness and futility, as expressed above by Josefa. And associated with these feelings is one of mixed desperation and restlessness, illustrated by the common complaint of having "desires to run away" (*deseos de seguir caminando*). A pattern of escape from problems or from oneself is built in to Puerto Rican life. The most common move when one is faced with severe marital, economic, or other difficulties is to go north to the United States. Recalcitrant teenagers are sent to Puerto Rico from the United States or the reverse; young women despairing of finding a mate will seek employment or advanced degrees in New York or another large Eastern city; divorced women search out another chance in life and better opportunities for employment; and men often abandon families by this route. Several depressed women said that they had tried a move to the States or were thinking about doing so as a solution to their marital or other relationship difficulties. Those who feel they are not able to escape seem to manifest more severe dysphoric moods and talk about suicide.

From these women we heard that flight from a situation they feel "tied to" offers them a means of control over their destinies. This is a kind of "control" that they despair of having over people on whom they have to depend. We reflected, privately, that by escaping, that is, by running away or committing suicide, they gain the male prerogative of power over their movements in life. However, of all the thirty cases that are the basis for our exploration of symbolic domains in depression and related life situations, only one revealed a history of suicide attempts.

Sonia

A doctor presented the case of

> Sonia, a thirty-year-old married woman with five children. Her initial complaints were that she felt "very depressed" and "desperate." Having left school at the

age of thirteen to live with her husband, she was ill prepared for the pain and difficulties married life held for her. When she became pregnant at age sixteen, her husband began running with other women. He drank a great deal and would hit her almost without excuse on returning from his nights out. He was especially abusive during her pregnancies. Seeking to ameliorate this situation, Sonia underwent sterilization following the birth of her last child, but his abuse not only continued but increased. She feels tremendously afraid of her husband and has been unable to confront him with her feelings. Instead she turns her anger on her children, beats them fiercely at times, but then feels terrible for having done so. Sonia especially takes her anger out on the oldest child, a boy of fourteen years, who has begun to talk about wanting to die. She planned to kill herself on three occasions and went to the health center to plead for barbiturates. She says that if she "cannot kill herself, she will go to the United States." After her husband gave her a venereal disease, Sonia felt that she could not "endure" any longer. She strategized how to avoid having sexual relations with him by staying up later and rising earlier but soon became worn out and very desperate. She again began to plan how she would kill herself.

All agreed that Sonia's situation is extreme in that the acknowledged authority and prerogatives of her husband, even though turned toward severe physical and psychological abuse, are accepted with such resignation. One Spiritist commented that there is often a time when a woman can no longer "hold it in" (*aguantar*). Women like Sonia who have little education and few skills feel (realistically) that they cannot get employment. They feel trapped in being unable to escape to another situation that will insure their personal survival and that of their children. They may get some emotional support from mothers or sisters, but these women are also likely to feel unempowered and actually have too few resources to provide economic assistance. We noted that this is the experiential backdrop to epidemiological studies that show that women who have jobs have fewer depressive symptoms than housewives (Brown and Harris, 1978; Roberts, 1981; Roberts and Roberts, 1982). One study of depression among Mexican Americans found that employment so ameliorated the expression of depressive symptomatology that women's rates of depression are the same as men's (rather than two times greater or more) when the women are employed (Roberts and Roberts, 1982).

The psychiatric epidemiological study described in the preceding chapter (Canino et al., 1987c; Canino et al., 1988) found that a full-time job protects against depression for both men and women, but a lack of education renders individuals more at risk. However, employment among *married* Puerto Rican women does not appear to protect against depression. If we reflect upon cases of depression in the present study, a clear message emerges: women who feel (and often actually are) entrapped by a difficult marital situation not only experience more severe depressive symptoms—often expressed as "I feel depressed and desperate"—but also are more likely to think about killing themselves.

A study of suicide attempts among Puerto Rican women in New York (Trautman, 1961) describes reports of subjective experience prior to the attempts. Women said, "I suddenly lost control of myself," "My mind went blank," and "I could not think anymore." These experiences are not uncommon among the depressed women in this book; they are linked with more general expressions about distress, such as *nervios*, *nerviosidad*, and *agitación*, but indicate an even greater depth of distressful feelings from which suicide is thought of as an escape. Trautman explicitly notes that among his patients there was a lack of awareness of, or fear of, death. He comments that "These patients were out of contact with reality, their rational thinking impaired, their behavior like people in a trance" (1961:99). The import of the experience of having one's thought processes taken over is explicitly recognized by the Spiritists and will be described later. They view "obsession" by a spirit as a major cause of complaints like "headache" and a general condition of distress they perceive as equivalent to "depression."

Trautman (1961) also commented that twenty-eight out of fifty women were affected by their menstrual cycles when they attempted suicide. Whereas he suggests that this contributed to a presuicidal state of excitability, if we view this from an interpretive perspective, it points again to the symbolic importance of women's reproductive systems in their experiences of distress. In Trautman's studies, approximately three-quarters of the women said quarrels with their husbands or lovers had precipitated their suicide attempts. Based on case material presented to the Project, I suggest that very basic feelings of self-worth are damaged by a woman's perception that she has been rejected by a mate, regardless of his role in the conflict and separation. Such feelings are greatly exacerbated when a woman feels she cannot achieve what she perceives to be the "highest" goal of women—motherhood. This is illustrated by the case of Milagros, described next, in which the mix of marital problems, feelings of loneliness, and early abandonment by her father are intensified by distress over her sterility.

Milagros

Anna H., Milagro's therapist, recounted:

> Milagros is thirty-seven and has been married nineteen years. She says that she is always "very nervous" and cannot "control herself." When she describes feeling "very sad and lonely," she begins to cry. She has problems with an adopted son, now 16 years old, whom she feels rejects her because she is not his natural mother. She reports that her husband doesn't understand her, and she has difficulties caring for a sick, eighty-nine-year-old aunt. Although "always

> nervous," this worsened when her mother died five years ago, because she "always lived with her," and they were "very attached" to one another.

Anna H. said that Milagros's father left her mother before she was born, and although she "knew" him, she never felt very much about him or his daughter from a subsequent relationship. However, the therapist commented that Milagros manifests a great deal of anxiety with regard to being unable to have children and is "excessively worried" about her adopted son's finding out that she is not his mother.

As mentioned earlier, we observed that many Puerto Ricans, especially women, feel it is impossible to avoid the affective impress of another's moods. Reactions to the moods of loved ones are particularly intense, as in the case of Milagros in relation to her adopted son. North Americans are invidiously contrasted with Puerto Ricans as being *frío* (cold), that is, nonreactive to emotions and feelings. Unfortunately, sensitivity toward others' feelings, which is generally given a positive value, also has a potentially negative side, a vaguely expressed feeling that one's self-boundaries are permeable to negative feelings expressed by other people—especially to feelings of anger or jealousy that are overtly directed at oneself.

As described previously, feeling "fearful" and having crying jags are the two most frequent complaints in Spiritist cases. It is explained that these complaints imply that a large component of the discourse on dysphoric affect is a fear for bodily survival—fear of serious illness or even death. Some mental health professionals had a similar perspective, as illustrated in the discussion of Delia's problems.

Delia

A psychiatrist told us:

> Delia is a young woman, twenty-two years of age, married to a younger man. The couple have two children. Delia works in a factory and is the family's provider. She reports that she has problems with her husband who doesn't work, causing her to have to work overtime to pay their bills. She is also distressed over conflict with her father. Delia originally presented at the mental health center with "palpitations," "insomnia," "little appetite," and "headaches" lasting seven months.

After carefully examining Delia, the psychiatrist said he concluded that she had no physical problems. However, in commenting about the case he repeated that both he and a consulting psychologist agreed that she was "dealing with her problems by channeling them through her body" and that she later might develop "hypertension," possibly "migraine" or "diabetes." Both thought that her situation must make her job very stressful but that she has so much responsibility that she cannot allow herself "to go crazy." She instead finds refuge in physical illness.

We observed that specific situations are mentioned in connection with suffering from headaches. One severely depressed woman, who also often suffers confusion, said that she cannot stand "violence" around her; her head "gets big and her chest feels oppressed" when her children fight. Moreover, headaches result when women have to control their feelings about their husbands' misdeeds, emotional outbursts, or abuse. The need to "hold in" distress as well as "hold up" in the face of personal suffering partly stems from economic and emotional dependency. We noted that it also seems to represent an attempt to live out culturally patterned expectations regarding what a "good" woman should do, that is, that she should be the stabilizing force in her marriage. Cohen's (1979) description of the case of a Latino woman who struggles to contain her disturbed emotions in the face of her husband's injunction that she should avoid thinking about their problems (under threat that he will leave her) perfectly illustrates this dilemma.

Headaches were explained by Spiritists to occur when the volume of problems "alters the clamor in your head." If not alleviated, they can lead to "depression." To prevent emotional distress one should bathe, rest, and "exorcise" (*despojar*) worries, that is, "get the disturbance out." It happens that a spirit who feels bad or sick looks for someone to help him. "Osmosis" occurs and the spirit "depresses" the person, changing happy responses to sad ones. The spirit then tries to isolate the victim because it wants to prevent her from receiving help; it is thus better able to control her. A spirit's invasion of the head or mind is referred to as *obsesión simple*, which several Spiritists equate with "depression." The implication is that the sufferer loses control over her emotions and feelings; her ability to reason or think clearly is blocked. This process is also given by Spiritists as an explanation of why some women manifest a host of complaints and are no longer able to "hold in" feelings of distress.

María

The way in which Spiritists relate serious illness to dysphoric mood is illustrated in the following report by a healer of the case of an eighteen-year-old girl.

> Three months before graduating from high school, María was hospitalized with tuberculosis. At the request of her mother, I visited her in the hospital and found her withdrawn, unwilling to eat or take medicine, completely refusing to cooperate with the doctors. When a person has a physical illness that isolates them from society, then they feel very depressed. I convinced her that if she submitted to a spiritual treatment, that I was sure she would get better. I gave her "magnetic passes" and counseled her. She took the medicines, ate, and got

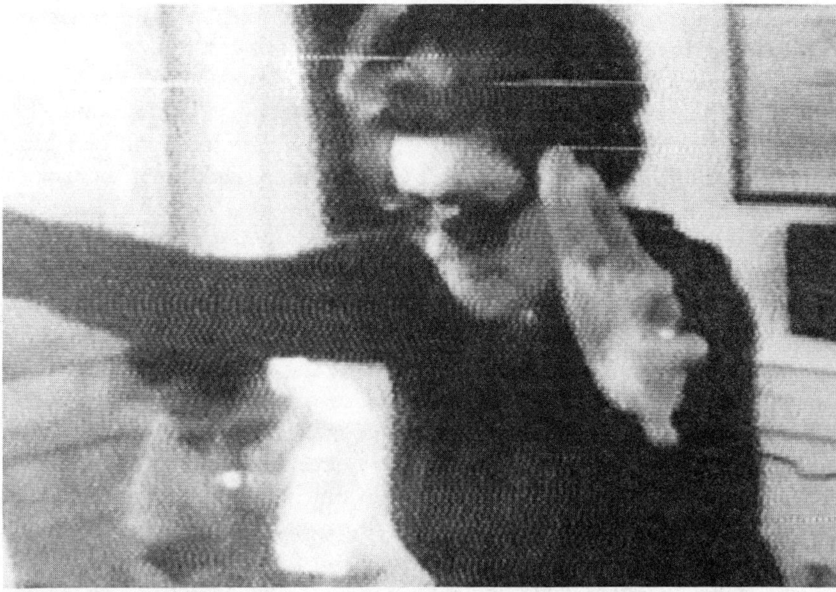

A medium works on a client to "lift off" a troublesome spirit.

> better. In fact, she attended sessions after she left the hospital and developed the faculties for "inspiration" and for hearing the spirits. She also finished her studies and married.

On being asked to explain the spiritual aspect of the illness, the healer replied, "Just as a human person can transmit [a disease] to you, a spirit also is able to transmit one, and even more so if the spirit died under these conditions." Then she explained that one's "soul" may have acquired an immunity in a past existence that provides a defense against the disease. And, "If you *think* you are tubercular, these thoughts, this negative energy that you yourself are producing. . . . is what you attract to you."

We observed that it seems clear that in the Spiritist view, physical illness and bodily complaints range along a continuum that begins with an individual's personal reactions to difficulty (including her spiritual history over many incarnations). The way in which she experiences dysphoric feelings can determine the appearance and seriousness of the complaints and whether and how they can be resolved. As one healer described: "You can become obsessed if you vibrate in affinity with the obsessor. Those who have the tendency to become angry frequently, to be violent or irate, have more capacity to become obsessed than the calm person." This explanation struck us as similar to a psychological theory of how personality traits relate to the expression of depressive symptoms, but it differs from this kind of explanation by focusing on how people relate to spirits who represent an integration of inner and outer forces that make up an individual's consciousness of self.

Two other differences between Spiritist and therapist views on "depression" that we especially noted were first, the previously mentioned difference in perspective on hallucinations versus visions. This subject will be treated in more detail in the next chapter. Here I will mention that the epidemiological researchers in Puerto Rico felt they had to revise Diagnostic Interview Schedule criteria for dysthymic disorder to include some "paranoid" features, visual experiences, auditory hallucinations, and tactile perceptions normally scored on the Diagnostic Interview Schedule as psychotic symptoms (Guevara Ramos et al., n.d.). Persons who are depressed but not psychotic talk about private visions and other sensations that cannot be accounted for by ordinary sensory validation. Such experiences are also reported by clinicians in the United States. (See Hoyt, 1980–1981, and Singer, 1976, among many others.)

We knew from experience that visionary experiences are a part of life for many Puerto Ricans who do not believe in Spiritism or other cults; visions are an accepted aspect of their culturally constituted environment. We discussed the fact that if accompanied by severe emotional distress, visions can be viewed as symbolic attempts to express special aspects of the content of the illness. In this, Spiritists share a perspective on visions with Freud, who said that visionary experiences revealed both the problem and its resolution. For Spiritists, visions are windows onto the patient's relations with the spirit world and its complex interpersonal arrangements. They either indicate that the client is "in development" of spiritual faculties or is undergoing a "test" in the process of spiritual evolution.

The second difference between therapist and Spiritist approaches to depression that we observed in their discussions regards the frequent complaint of clients of Spiritists that they are in a state of "mental confusion." This complaint is commonly associated both with "sadness" and with conflict between the "moral and material" aspects of life, that is, moral dilemmas. The case of Carmen illustrates the Spiritist approach. For them, "confusion" is different from the psychiatric definition as "indecisiveness," "slow thinking," or "difficulty in concentrating" (APA, 1980).

Carmen

A Spiritist healer recounted:

> Carmen is thirty-two years of age, unmarried, a practicing Catholic, and employed by the government. She lives with her parents with whom she says she had "good relations." Two brothers have married and moved away. She is healthy but confirms that she is always sad, especially in relation to her mother.
>
> I "saw" [that is, had a *videncia*] that Carmen's parents generously provide for this young woman but do not show warmth or love. But man doesn't live on

bread alone. The conflict in this woman is due to the fact that her parents tie her to them through religious principles that demand strong respect. Carmen is unable to participate in life as she desires, to go out with men, dance, or smoke. She has been held back from seeking her own life and the love for which she longs.

Key Events and Life Situations of Depressed Women

Let me now highlight aspects of the descriptions above and summarize the thirty cases on which this chapter is based. Women diagnosed as "depressed" and those with parallel complaints treated by Spiritists appear to be most commonly affected by three kinds of negative life experiences: rejection or abandonment by a parent, which is especially severe when a mother dies or leaves; the threat of or actual abandonment by a mate and fears about survival without him; and problems related to the capacity for motherhood, frequently a result of reproductive system malfunctions. In addition to these prominent experiences, there are others that are less frequent. For example, we recalled the two young Spiritist clients with reactive "depressions" to serious illness (and other events) that they reported had kept them from getting on with their life goals of mating and motherhood. In the cases of three other women, two seen by Spiritists and one seen by a therapist, this problem was expressed in another way: these women said they felt blocked from achieving their desired life goals by having to care for aged parents whom they were "tied" to.

We encountered a number of cases in which women felt abandoned by a parent. The mother of one woman left her as a small girl with her grandparents in order to remarry and another mother died when her daughter was a year old. Many also felt affectively distant from parents who did not abandon them. Several women raised without fathers suffered crises when their mothers died; they tended to have prior histories of "feeling rejected" before they presented for treatment.

We noted that most depressed women do not spontaneously mention past relations with their families of origin but instead focus on current family situations as sources of distress. These women suffer mainly from fears of abandonment by their husbands or mates or from reactions to having been deserted by prior mates. These cases are much like those described by Torres Matrullo (1982) of Puerto Rican women in New York; she sees the origins of distress in these cases as closely associated with cultural prescriptions for desirable womanly behavior.

It seemed to us that many depressed women, whether or not employed, were unable to imagine themselves without a mate. They preferred to struggle with extremely difficult marital situations rather than live alone and be seen by others as lacking worth as a woman. It is as if they felt they were not whole; they required a relationship with a man to feel worthy. The reader is reminded of an earlier discussion about how concepts of the feminine self develop in relation to overt denigration of single women. There are suspicions that such women are sexually "unnatural," and there is covert stigmatization of women who divorce their husbands, although this is changing as more women independently pursue professions and accept divorce as a necessary evil.

We observed that if a mother or child has died, women express feelings of abandonment that remain intense over years. Nine out of the thirty women whose cases form the substantive material for this chapter complained that they grievously missed mothers or children who had died some time ago, from eleven months to more than ten years earlier. Most gave this as the reason for their sadness or loneliness. Two women whose husbands had died were also sad and felt abandoned, yet they did not speak of the absence of their husbands as a cause of their dysphoria.

Concerns about sterility, menopause, abortion (spontaneous), and being unable to have another child reflect the fact that a capacity for motherhood is central to self-concepts about "the good woman." Assessment of feminine self-worth is directly affected by reproductive problems or failures, even when a husband has had a vasectomy. Two women diagnosed as being in psychotic depressive episodes felt that their genitals were being attacked by an outside force. We reflected that these sensations could even be considered "rational," because abusive husbands deeply attack a woman's sense of self-worth. The frequent hallucinations or visions of threatening men experienced by women diagnosed as suffering from "major depression" seem to have a similar meaning. They could be explained as projections of male threats to female self-worth.[3]

With regard to those women with dysphoria who feel tied to parents, I have observed that some Puerto Rican parents attempt to keep one child home to care for them in their old age. A daughter is the usual choice because sons are relatively free from parental restrictions from late childhood onward. (However, I also knew parents who kept a homosexual son close to them.) Sometimes the chosen daughter will marry but continue to live with her parents, and in other cases, having a child outside of wedlock will reinforce the woman's dependency upon her parents. Seriously depressed daughters seem unable to make even those types of adjustments in the face of heavy parental demands for their attention.

Treatment Strategies for Depression: Therapists and Spiritists Compared

In Chapters 3 and 4 I compared how therapists, doctors, and Spiritists work with patients. Here I will describe and compare notions and interventions specific to cases of women diagnosed as depressed. In the large sample of 131 cases of women diagnosed as suffering "dysthymic disorder," the most frequent mental health treatments were individual therapy (76 percent); supportive therapy (20 percent); and drug therapy: type of medication unspecified (27 percent), Elavil (24 percent), Mellaril (18 percent), and Norpramil (8 percent). Patients diagnosed with major depression generally received the same treatments, with the exception that they rarely received individual psychotherapy.

In the Spiritist cases of depression, spirits who invade are often interpreted to be potential *guías*; clients are told that the *causa* spirit molesting them is a sign of their being "in development" as mediums. At one session, a woman who felt lonely and cried a great deal was told by an *Espiritista*, "Do not cry. That spirit is with you and you are no longer alone." We were present when Rosa was treated and observed how spirit support is attained through "development."

Rosa

> Rosa was the first to be called to the table at that session. Eight *videncias* were reported to her by the mediums at the table, who also plied her with questions after each *videncia*. She was told about and confirmed a long list of complaints: "feelings of desperation," "nervousness," "headaches that are not too severe," "heart and chest vibrations," "fatigue," "tiredness," and difficulty falling asleep at night yet excessive sleepiness during the day. In addition, her "eyes smart," she "feels sad yet is unable to cry," her "ears itch," she is "bewildered" (*cabeza aturdida*), and she "feels like running away." One of the *videncias* imaged a spirit who brings her "powers" that she should expand upon.
>
> Rosa confessed that she formerly practiced as a healer but stopped because of lack of faith. A medium who finally took Rosa's spirit *causa* into her body told Rosa that he (the spirit) is always with her and makes her do "bad works." It is he who causes all of these complaints. The spirit is a "heavy black man" with a swollen face who died "obsessed" and makes Rosa fearful. She is told to pray more, have faith and love. She must pray to help this spirit, whose motive is vengeance so great that he doesn't want to let go of her. The spirit in the possessed medium says, "If you are guilty, I am more so. Give yourself to God."

We knew that the ritual act is aimed at getting rid of the molesting spirit's influence, but the content of the spirit's message seemed directed toward the strong sense of wrongdoing that Rosa expressed. He mirrored her feelings of guilt yet also took the blame for her deeds as well as her symptoms. The implication is that as a spirit worker she had carried out bad works and was now reaping the reward of a divided soul. The mediums at this session probed for all possible complaints commonly associated with depression, including asking Rosa if she had attempted suicide. Their interventions in her case were directed at personal transformation as well as insisting that she develop

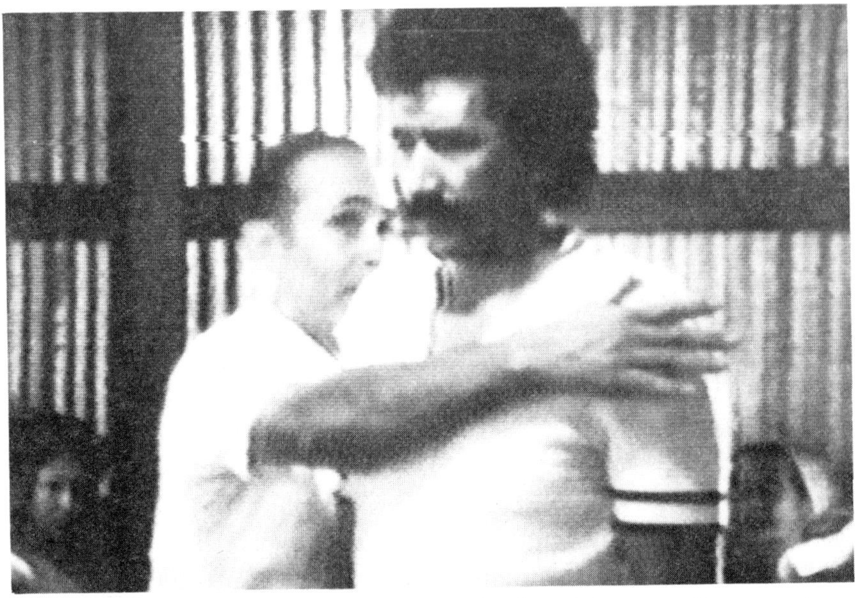

A medium attempts to "strip off" a spirit that has been blocking a client's emotions.

a sense of dedication to an altruistic, God-serving life as a mediumistic healer, assisted by the acquisition of new spirit guides. (This was one of the few occasions when guilt was specifically mentioned.)

The case of Milagros (who felt rejected by her adopted son), described earlier in this chapter, was presented to the joint review session by a mental health worker-psychologist and commented on by Spiritist healers. The psychologist's approach to therapy was based upon both a theory of personality development and notions about the role of stressful events in triggering emotional disorder. She noted that Milagros had always been nervous, but her condition worsened when her mother died some five years before. At that time Milagros presented for help at the psychiatric hospital. She "hardly knew her father, and now her mother was dead." This perspective emphasized her aloneness in the world.

The therapist offered Milagros "supportive therapy" in order to help her "understand her mother's death," which she described as the focus of her work with Milagros. She also said she was working on problems having to do with lack of communication in Milagros's marriage and Milagros's fear of rejection by her adopted son. The therapist's goals with Milagros were aided by establishing a relationship of confidence between them, which was meant to allow Milagros the comfort of venting her feelings. The therapist also felt that she should attempt to do family therapy with Milagros, with a particular focus on the marital relationship. She hoped that through understanding the problems of adolescence Milagros could rid herself of worries about her adopted son's lack of affection. In order to counter the lonely feelings associated with Milagros's mother's death, she suggested that Milagros participate in church or volunteer activities and expand her social arena so as not to focus all of her feelings on her nuclear family. These moves were said to be aimed at lessening Milagros's feelings of isolation through enlarging her social networks.

Although Milagros had been seen on a weekly basis for about four months, she currently was on an "open, come-as-needed appointment." Later the therapist reported that Milagros's complaints were less severe, but she had not yet informed her adopted son of his true status, and her husband had not come in for treatment.

One of the Spiritists disagreed with the therapist's focus on Milagros's mother's death, saying that she felt that Milagros's main problem was fear of "abandonment" by her son. She thought the direction of treatment should be to give Milagros a sense of "spiritual security" with regard to her place as the mother of this boy, justified by the fact that she had raised him. Milagros must be made to see that "death is the most natural thing in the world" and we have to "pass through this change." This reflects the Spiritists' positive stance toward death as transformation rather than finality. Another Spiritist healer insisted that Milagros was not only concerned with the problems she expressed but also with "knowing herself." "But it is as if she is floating."

It appeared to us that both kinds of healer were pointing to a quality of "motherlessness" in Milagros, with regard to both her separation through death from a mother on whom she was very dependent emotionally and her being thwarted in her desire to "mother" her son. (One might speculate that the image of "floating" is opposite to a sense of being grounded in the earth, the "mother" of us all.)

As might be expected given the type of training in psychology these therapists had had, they usually approached depression looking through cognitive and behavioral lenses. Thus they would find a direction in the way in which a patient was maladjusted. They then dealt with the maladjustment by reasoning with the patient or by giving her behavioral prescriptions aimed at changes in attitude and interpersonal relations. Help was given within a supportive, trusting relationship, which therapists worked hard to achieve. In contrast, the Spiritists generally viewed problems such as those experienced by Milagros as existential concerns. Their usual perspective on chronic, severe emotional problems in people who were not functionally disabled was that such symptoms were painful opportunities for self-knowledge and spiritual transformation. For them it was necessary for Milagros to "learn how to live," that is, to find meaning in life. These two perspectives are very different in scope as well as method, with the Spiritists tending to view depression as even more serious than do the therapists. Torres-Matrullo's (1982) success in using Beck's Cognitive Behavioral Treatment with Puerto Rican women may be due to the fact that it incorporates aspects of both approaches, because it seeks to correct what are labeled as "faulty assumptions" about the self and about how women should behave.

Cases diagnosed as "major depression with psychotic features" are commonly treated by psychiatrists in mental health clinics with both antidepressant and antipsychotic medication as well as brief hospitalization. Spiritists may view delusions or hallucinations as spirit evidence but usually agree that both psychiatric and spiritual treatment are necessary in such cases. In regard to Carmen, for example, they said they saw "*tristeza en el alma*" (sadness in her soul) and a state of "mental confusion." They suggested that she attend thirty-six sessions over three months (three per week). The spirit molesting her was judged to be "very tenacious." In discussing this case, a psychologist remarked that mental illness is too difficult for Spiritists to treat, because they know so little about the mind. An *Espiritista* retorted that we are all dominated by concern for our physical bodies, but "our spirits are ruining our bodies instead of allowing them to be the vehicle of our spirit's progress."

Although they believe spirits cause depressive syndromes, we observed Spiritists to regularly pay attention to how spirits affected a client's body. For example, one woman treated at a *centro* was described as "very thin, with a bony face and sunken eyes." "She looked very needy." She was admonished by a medium: "You have a body and you have a spirit. Just as you look for sustenance, you need to look for food for your spirit, such as prayers for conformity, resignation, love, and kindness in relationships." Later her progress was measured by a weight gain of forty pounds after five visits, and it was noted that her demeanor was now one of happiness. This client was encouraged to stay in psychiatric treatment until discharged by the doctor.

In contrast, the mental health workers tended to measure change almost exclusively in terms of behavior, especially in terms of the ways in which a woman carried out her roles of wife and mother.

Conclusion

I have explored dysphoria and depression as syndromes interpreted as distress, labeled as psychiatric disorder in mental health clinics and as *obsesión simple* in Spiritist *centros*. As might be expected, the types of complaints expressed by depressed women in Puerto Rico are similar to those described in psychiatric manuals for other populations. However, they differ from descriptions of depression in the United States in terms of interpretations given to these complaints by both sufferers and healers, in terms of their relative frequencies, and in terms of the patterning of specific situations with which they are associated. In this and the following three chapters I take the approach of "cultural analysis," which is that the content and expression of dsyphoric or any types of feelings can only be understood within the context of a set of culturally structured interactions that give them meaning (Schieffelin, 1985). This approach is actually very similar to that of the Spiritists, who bring out the "inner" experiences of clients in relation to their feelings of distress. They interpret clients' emotions and feelings as integral to a web of human and spirit relationships that has become unbalanced or damaged, resulting in loss of control over emotions and feelings.

The core symptoms of depressive disorders, according to the diagnostic psychiatric manual, are "dysphoric mood, usually depression, or loss of interest or pleasure in all or almost all usual activities and pastimes" (APA, 1980). Considering the narratives in this chapter, it seems that these "core" symptoms are not central elements in discourse about dysphoria and distress in women diagnosed as depressed in Puerto Rico—that is, in the initial presentations and discourse between women as patients and their therapists or between clients and Spiritist healers. Somatic complaints appear to be much more prominent; moreover, they point to a multiplicity of social and psychological problems and stressful life events. It is difficult to measure some symptoms listed as associated with the principle ones in the diagnostic manuals, such as feeling one's energy reduced or decreased interest in life or loss of the capacity to enjoy life, in a culture that mandates people to express feelings of an enjoyment of life, of an energetic interest in people and events, and so on. Self-reports are essential to securing this information, with patients formulating both the complaints and the judgments. If we examine the situations of women as patients and clients in Puerto Rico, we find that discourse is most frequently about somatic complaints, which symbolically reflect experience about their bodies and their bodies' needs in relation to closely associated self-concepts. "Nervousness" as a chief complaint in depressed women has a large psychological component; but it is even closer to a notion like "psyche-soma," the *periespiritu* of the Spiritists, the connection between mind and body.

Therapists focus mainly on behavioral outcomes of dysphoric mood and emotions, but Spiritists seem to highlight changes in attitude and self-concept, even though these are detected indirectly. Guilt is mentioned infrequently, but contemplation of suicide as escape is fairly common.

Another cultural difference is that loss of sexual drive is only referred to obliquely when women healers or mental health workers discuss cases among themselves and is rarely expressed as a complaint by their patients or clients. This reflects the high value placed on privacy of sexual life by these women and a lack of emphasis on their sexual motivations as important to sexual relations. And we again note that they are far more preoccupied with reproductive capacity than with sexual satisfaction. As described in many studies (Canino, 1982) and in literature by women about women (Vega and

Lugo Filippi, 1981), the Virgin holds a much higher place as a self-symbol than does Venus, although this might be changing among younger women.

Notes

1. Harwood (1977) discusses the prominent role of gossip among Puerto Rican neighbors in New York.

2. This is the case in which a woman accused her husband of securing a bad spell that affected her genitals and made her feel "dead in life," without a "spirit," and as if "in another world."

3. As discussed in prior chapters, "to hallucinate" is not a concept that has meaning for Spiritist believers, who interpret "nonreal," nonpresent phenomena to be visions of spirits that may or may not connote illness or emotional distress.

8

Madness and Schizophrenia

While a great many persons classified as schizophrenic do indeed report hallucinations, recent research has led to serious questioning about what is actually meant by this phenomenon. Is the patient really hearing voices or seeing images, or is he possibly misinterpreting his private fantasies, assuming that they come from the outside mainly because he has listened so little to his own consciousness in childhood? Most schizophrenic patients do not show a great vividness of inner fantasy or even great complexity in their hallucinations.

—Jerome Singer, *Daydreaming and Fantasy*

The Meaning and Fear of *Locura* (Craziness)

Over twenty-five years ago, just prior to the initiation of the Community Mental Health Center Program by the Puerto Rican Department of Health, Rogler and Hollingshead (1961, 1965) collected folk theories of mental illness from a group of people with low incomes. "*Locos*," according to their informants, are given to sudden acts of violence and to the most extreme of bizarre behaviors. They are dirty, dress inappropriately, and generally behave in ways contrary to those of "decent" people. Considerable fear of locos was expressed. An exception was the *loco tranquilo*, who lives on the streets of *barrios* or in business districts of most towns and is tolerated as a kind of town jester. I remember a "quiet crazy man" who lived in the streets of Old San Juan for many years. Dressed in a World War II army jacket complete with campaign ribbons, he burlesqued passersby and the authorities but was supported by local businessmen. Such street people are almost always male. Mentally ill women are usually kept at home or cared for in institutions.

At the time that Rogler carried out his study, there was only one public psychiatric hospital in Puerto Rico. The hospital had fifteen hundred beds. It had generally poor facilities, and its administrators had just begun to think about more modern treatment of mental illness. Moreover, it was always crowded and understaffed. Most families cared for their mentally ill relatives by locking them up in special rooms or shacks adjacent to their homes, usually freeing them during periods between violent episodes. This was still the case in the early 1960s, during the inauguration of the Community Mental Health Center Act in the United States. This kind of treatment is now much rarer, given the expansion and updating of mental health care services, including a full-scale community mental health program and anti-psychotic drugs that assist in maintaining chronically mentally ill people in their community settings.

There is still great fear among many people of being labeled a loco, which not only carries great social stigma but also an underlying notion that the condition is incurable. "Nerves" or "nervousness" are terms often used by patients diagnosed as mentally ill to talk about their conditions. Families of women in the present study who have been diagnosed as psychiatrically ill, the patients themselves, and even the doctors when referring to their mentally ill relatives almost always talk about "nervousness" or "nerves." As mentioned earlier, to "have nerves" can refer to a serious condition, roughly parallel to what psychiatry calls psychosis, and implies that it runs in family lines. Despite some knowledge among both lay people and psychiatric patients of psychiatric models of mental disorder, many still express an underlying fear that their nervous condition will result in their becoming a "crazy person." Such fears are especially prevalent among those actually diagnosed as suffering schizophrenia; few appear to have a realistic view of what psychiatry means by this disease label.

None of the women in this study diagnosed as schizophrenic (or with other diagnoses for that matter) uses the word *loco* or *locura* to describe her own condition or her experience of it. Surprisingly, the term is rare in all of the extensive data gathered in this project, with the exception of its use by Spiritist healers who describe how certain spirits affect people by "having them crazy." This refers more to an experience of erratic, uncontrolled behavior than a condition diagnosable as mental illness. "Loco" may also be used to describe someone whose actions are erratic or bizarre, a popular reference to crazy-like behavior in normal people.

Spiritist Notions of Madness

If euphoria characterizes the public dimension of the Puerto Rican ethos, "madness," as a term representing extreme distress and out-of-control behavior, is at the very core of the Puerto Rican ethos. In contrast, the concept of being "depressed" seems to be a genre of experience imposed upon indigenous Puerto Rican concepts. To be "crazy" is a deeply feared state that can easily be imagined; it appears to be an imagined reality for almost everyone. This in part explains why spiritual explanations are so popular among both believers in Spiritism and those mentally ill people and their families who find their way to *centros*.[1] Resort to Spiritism can be even more important to some people who are not psychiatrically ill but who fear that their experiences of spontaneous alterations of consciousness mean that they are becoming crazy.

Complaints about the "mind" are frequently expressed by Spiritists and their clients. These complaints are presented by 16 percent of the people diagnosed by therapists as schizophrenic. The most frequent complaint is that the "mind leaves" or goes blank (*se le va la mente, se le queda en blanco*). The mind can also be "disturbed," "molested," "stalled," "turned over," "turned around," "running on," or "warped." All of these conditions are attributed by mediums to spirit influences on the way the mind (or brain) affects behavior. Whereas therapists may describe a patient as speaking incoherently, with interrupted thought process and impaired memory, Spiritist healers say that "some spiritual being is interlocked with or hooked onto" the individual. As in Spiritist explanations of depression, such people are also said to be "obsessed" but to a even greater degree that "perturbs" the mind and causes it to malfunction.

According to the Spiritists, obsession by a "perennial thought" that invades the mind can also have this effect. Those affected have an impossibly large "emotional burden" or "tension" that renders them vulnerable to spirits, who then become attached to them. Fear is a principal contributor to this state, yet symptoms of "nervousness" may not affect the mind to any extreme degree for years until one day the person suffers a "nervous shock." This occurred in Juana's case, described later in the discussion on hallucinations. Juana attributed her complaints to her father's coming home drunk, knocking on her bedroom door, and asking about her mother. She was always unable to return to sleep. However, when he came one night and was particularly insistent, she became extremely distressed and emotional and later said she "saw a serpent." However, this was not the worst possible case of "obsession"; "persecution by an invisible enemy" can lead to homocide or suicide. The "enemy" is a spirit sent by a living person or someone known in a former existence who is not simply making a mistake by impacting the life and body of the victim but wishes her (or him) harm.

Some Spiritists say that there are two types of *locura*. One is the result of lesions in the brain and is referred to as "physical madness"; the other is called *locura espiritual* and stems from ignorance of "*Quién soy yo?*" that is, not knowing who one is. For example, an *Espiritista* observed at one of the Project's meetings that a symptomatic schizophrenic girl's own spirit was totally out of her body; she was "subjugated." This notion is similar to that of demonic possession, except that (in most cases) the dominating spirit is not evil in nature and may even be a potential *guía* of a client in development. The result of the "obsession" by a spirit is that the person doesn't know herself or even *who* is behaving. She experiences great inner conflict with regard to who is motivating her actions. We commented that these concepts are similar to psychological theories of psychosis that view its cause or dynamics as an overwhelming of the ego, defined as the control center of the personality. (See Crapanzano and Garrison, 1979.) Spirits of living people are thought of as neither external nor internal to the personality; they are individual entities who endow the body (*la materia*) with self-knowledge and life force. One's own spirit can be completely displaced by invasive spirit beings who take over the body, causing bizarre behavior and distress.

Hostility or aggressiveness, a frequent complaint that we observed, has two main associations in the experiences of schizophrenic women. The most poignant are feelings (often reflecting fact) of total rejection by one's family. Failure to identify with one's mother and thus achieve a feminine identity is also common. The case of Herminia, desribed next, illustrates how a woman's entire life may be colored by a premorbid disordered personality, in part shaped by the hostile acts of her parents. There are no records that could have told us whether Herminia was born with organic defects that accounted for her autistic-like behavior as a child. From what she said it appears, however, that she had experienced hostile feelings and acts during most of her life, with the result that she often feels and displays hostility toward others.

Herminia

A social worker who presented Herminia's case told us:

> Herminia is fifty-seven years old. She lives alone but participates in Project Hope, a program for the elderly. She was one of ten siblings in a poor, rural family. She says that she feels "lonely," "ashamed," and "doesn't much care" about herself or "want anything from anybody since no one cares for her." She has nightmares and difficulty sleeping. According to her therapist, Herminia manifests "violent depressive states, pulls her hair, and throws herself against the wall as if to kill herself," behavior that apparently began in childhood. Herminia reports her symptoms to have begun after she once hit herself particularly hard.
>
> Herminia describes relations with her family as very poor; her siblings are hostile and never have spoken with her. She traces their attitudes to her father who "would not allow them to communicate" with her. When Herminia was five, she remembers being sent away from her home. Her mother apparently did not object because she submitted to Herminia's father in all things. She was then raised in institutions and in various foster homes for several years but was subsequently hospitalized. She walked out of the hospital at eighteen years of age. While there, she acquired a fourth grade education.
>
> Once having left the hospital, Herminia immediately found a man with whom to live. But by nineteen years of age she had been raped by various men. Over the next years she lived with five other men and bore three sons. Two were taken from her and placed in foster homes, but she cared for one boy, who left

her in his early teens to live with one of the men whom he knew as a child. Project Hope initially found her an apartment to share with this son, but they "hated" each other so much that they separated after only three months. The son reported that Herminia had punished him cruelly when he was a child.

Herminia says that she believes in Spiritism; she sees "images" who call her and talk with her. However, she feels sharp pains in her head when this happens. She refuses antipsychotic medication, saying that she wants to be as "free and wild as when I was born." When offered tranquilizers she also refuses because she "wants to function like a normal person, without any medication." A devout Catholic, she has been helped by the church and one priest in particular. Herminia's participation in Project Hope resulted in her being socialized to eat with utensils and becoming much calmer when interacting with other clients. She especially likes to attend parties where she feels "freer."

Presented by her therapist as a "chronic schizophrenic," Herminia's behavior is often so deviant that few can tolerate her. The persistent social worker working with Herminia at Project Hope told us that she insisted that Herminia conform to certain basic rules. This social worker was so sympathetic to Herminia's plight that Herminia responded favorably by behaving in a more cooperative and less aggressive way. Yet her usual response to new people and situations is one of immediate hostility, which seemed to us to be rather easily accounted for by her early experiences in life.

We noted that the taboo on open expression of aggressive behavior is so strong that it is difficult to actually observe "hostility" in women's behavior. It does occur in underground ways, as described in Chapter 5, as malicious gossip, witchcraft plots, and accusations. At the extreme of emotional distress, open violence can occur, most often directed against a rival for one's husband's love. An angry wife might damage his mistress's car or (more rarely) confront her with a verbal attack, which might lead to blows. However, as we often observed, deviant, out-of-control behavior, especially in women, arouses considerable fear. We knew that the primary focus of socialization of both male and female children is to inculcate respect and obedience; and parents are extremely distressed when children do not conform to their and society's expectations. People who behave violently or hostilely are referred to as "animals" to differentiate them from "educated" people who exhibit more passive human qualities. Nevertheless, I have often observed that "animal-like" behavior appears to be close to the surface in many people (although perhaps more in men than in women) and apparently experienced by them as difficult to control.

We reflected upon the notion that the association between mental illness and hostile feelings is not fortuitous. A failure to identify early in any way with one's mother, especially in a society where the mother role is both exalted and strongly urged upon women, leaves a daughter with a permanent sense of unrelatedness. Psychological theories based on ideas about "object relations"—that is, how well a mother has mirrored her child's sense of self when the child was eighteen months to three years old—explain in fine detail how the child comes to suffer a narcissistic wound, permanent damage to her sense of self-esteem (Kohut, 1971; Guntrip, 1969).

The phenomenology of the experience of narcissism is patently clear in Herminia's remarks about herself, shaped in her case by the sad experience of being abused as a child. Her words express the "self-hate, hunger, secret longing, and lack of bestowing warmth, exactly the workings of the deep-seated envy that controls the narcissistic character's inner life. This state of envy is a result of rejecting the Self" (Schwartz-Salant, 1982:24). What is called "schizophrenia" is a mental illness typified by extreme perceptual, cognitive, and behavioral disorders that seem to cover over and mask narcissistic wounds. Personality characteristics that are precursors of schizophrenia (in addition to a genetic predisposition for the disease or prenatal brain damage causing emotional and behavioral deficits) include the early inability to achieve self-object differentiation and a basic failure to acquire a sense of personal identity (Werner, 1985). Given the cultural ambience of Puerto Rico, the failure of a woman to identify with her mother (and her mother to receive her as a desirable person) is especially serious. To speculate, the consequences may reach beyond the already difficult effects of narcissistic wounding on the personality because such a failure directly interferes with the core of a Puerto Rican woman's self-worth—motherhood.

Hostile and aggressive behaviors, intertwined with desire for love and approval through a relationship with mother and motherhood, and failure to achieve an identity or sense of self are all illustrated in the case of Celia.

Celia

A mental health technician met Celia in the day hospital program of the CMHC; Celia had been diagnosed as schizophrenic. Clara H. recounted:

> Born in Puerto Rico and raised in New York, at sixteen she was in her second year of high school and pregnant. Celia asked her mother's permission to marry the father, a man several years her senior. However, she soon found that he was a drug addict. Some months after they married, he began to hit her, take her money, and disappear for long periods. Observing the situation worsening, Celia's mother decided that her daughter had to divorce this man and moved her, the baby, and the furnishings of her apartment into her parents' home. Although Celia followed her mother's dictates, she claimed it was against her will since she had been set up to believe that the man would be a "bad husband." She persisted in saying that she loved him and wanted to "make a home" with him. Celia said she accepted her mother's decision at the time because she "never had the opportunity to make decisions" for herself. Shortly after the

> divorce was final, Celia suffered her first psychotic episode. She was hospitalized at Bellevue Hospital in New York for twenty days.
>
> During Celia's hospital stay, her mother was advised that her daughter was not capable of caring for her child. She gave the little girl to Celia's brother and his wife, who later adopted her. Celia became enraged when discharged from the hospital but was again unable to protest her mother's actions. She became pregnant again, but this time the young man did not want to marry her. After giving birth, Celia fell into another "crisis," was again hospitalized—for a week this time. Again her mother took the baby away from her and gave the boy to Celia's sister, who adopted him. Apparently Celia's mother did not want to care for these grandchildren and said she felt overburdened by having to care for Celia. The same sequence of events was again repeated when Celia was nineteen and twenty-three years of age. However, her mother consented to keep the last child, who was two years old when we first encountered Celia, by then twenty-six years of age. At the time of the last child's birth, Celia consented to the "operation" [tubal ligation]. A disabled sister, the youngest of her siblings, takes care of this last child. When Celia saw me [her present therapist] for the first time, she asserted that what she wanted most was to recover her first three children and have all of her children in a home with her, in a house separated from her mother.

We noted that the history of Celia's illness and of her mother's responses to her behavior and stated needs seems typical of the way in which mothers can dominate their daughters' lives by preempting their autonomy and their right to independent decision making. A Spiritist to whom Celia was eventually referred by her therapist (I will describe later how they shared Celia's treatment) remarked that during her first visit to Celia's mother's home she had the "impression" that Celia's mother's attitude toward her was one of "I will do whatever I want to, and you shut up." The healer suggested that Celia, as do all human beings, has a "mission in this world, a place and certain things to do." Another Spiritist maintained that "if one doesn't know oneself, then it is like it is with machines. . . . [They] chew and chew and when they are empty there is the machinist who has returned to fill them again. This is what has occurred in the past with this sister. Everything that she has done is through the machinist, who is her mother." A therapist commenting on the case related this way of conceptualizing Celia's problems to the notion that "autonomy is the most important thing [we can have]; the greater one's autonomy, the better their self-esteem. When we speak about self-esteem, it is how one sees oneself in relation to the world." All seemed to be suggesting that Celia's difficulties were directly associated with psychological abuse from her mother, who had prevented Celia from realizing herself as an independent entity.

A third Spiritist healer added:

> A mother should not attack her daughter, nor the daughter her mother; respect is warranted. . . . The position of Spiritism is that they were enemies in another existence. No doubt, in this moment we understand that relations have deteriorated to a point where daughter and mother are not seeing each other as daughter and mother but instead as enemies. Our position would be to establish communication [between them] and that they should begin to ventilate their hostilities within the framework of an understanding, that is, where guilt won't be generated. . . . The mother offers a series of rejections, of lack of recognition, and of hostility towards the daughter. In turn the daughter relates back with rejection, hate, and agressivity. A moment arrives when they become aware, and the mother says, "It is you, my dear daughter." [She replies,] "Yes, my beloved mother." The relation changes automatically; they enter into real contact with each other.

This last statement, illustrating how Spiritists view mothers and daughters, made it clear to us that Spiritists believe in the awakening of awareness of what they view as basic and important feelings of love between intimate others, once distressing feelings of anger have been allowed to flow freely. This is a highly unusual suggestion because of the heavy proscription against anger in the family setting.

Celia's condition (according to the Spiritist healer who subsequently became Celia's mentor describing the first time she saw Celia) was typical of a flagrant, severe psychotic episode. When, at the suggestion of the therapist who had seen Celia in day care, her mother sought a pass to take Celia (then again hospitalized) to the *centro*, the psychiatrist at the psychiatric hospital at first denied it, saying that Celia's case was one of "serious aggression." Celia had been observed to regularly engage in fist fights with other patients and run naked through the corridors. But her mother was pained at the sight of her daughter in "conditions that were like those of wild animals." Celia's mother was able to wangle a fifteen-day pass for her daughter; however, she took her back to the hospital in six days and never got her to the *centro* because Celia became uncontrollably aggressive and threatened to kill all of the members of her family.

When Celia finally did appear at the *centro* on a second pass, she had red and swollen eyes, the result of blows sustained from fighting in the hospital. When questioned by a medium, Celia said that she "had to get up at five o'clock AM to tend the cows." Then she rapidly changed the subject, saying that she was "pregnant with twins on one side and bricks on the other." In rapid succession, she told the Spiritists and assembled believers that she had sexual relations with her husband (who was far away), and at night she saw animals and her husband on the wall. She said that she had been raped when she was ten years old, and that was why she was pregnant. Further, she accused her mother of murdering her children each time they were born. She then gave a false name.

The Spiritist healer's only response was to place Celia in the center of a circle formed by all present at the session, where she was then given "magnetic passes." In addition, two mediums attempted to heal Celia by using their "body energy." She was described as "getting better" in the second of four sessions to which she was brought during her second and third fifteen-day passes from the psychiatric hospital. A research assistant on the Project visited the *centro* during the fourth session Celia attended. She noted that Celia was able to give "appropriate" answers to a number of questions, including the date, and that her affect was also "appropriate." Apparently, Celia was no longer in a psychotic state. (Whether this was due to the Spiritists' treatment or a process of spontaneous remission cannot be demonstrated. However, Celia said she believed it was because of her work with the healers.)

Perspectives on Hallucinations, Delusions, and Visions

We present these last details on Celia's madness in order to provide the reader with some idea of the nature of psychotic behavior. From the viewpoint of the Spiritists who saw her, Celia was in an "apparently nervous crisis, outside of reality." They said that "her own spirit was outside her body," "it was totally outside," "subjugated." Such a person is subject to the effects of backward spirits and has no spirit guide—she is unable to be aware of one, because she is unable to know herself. The onsets of such crises are considered *pruebas* (tests) that must be experienced if the person is to "develop spirit powers at any time in the future."

The psychiatric records and comments by the mental health professionals showed that Celia manifested "delusions," "visual hallucinations," "incoherence, illogical thinking, and loosening of associations." Various researchers into clinical phenomena, such as Manfred Bleuler, have pointed out that schizophrenic mechanisms are found in normal people, but schizophrenics cannot distinguish between the realities of their inner and outer worlds (Lehmann and Cancro, 1985). Both "delusion" and "hallucination," coined from Latin words by Lavater (1572), refer to "an idea or belief to which nothing real corresponds." DSMIIIR (APA, 1987) requires that delusions, hallucinations, or other cognitive disturbances be present for the diagnosis of a schizophrenic disorder, but it must be noted that the *Comprehensive Textbook of Psychiatry* (Kaplan and Saddock, 1985) cautions that the diagnosis does not rest on the presence of delusions or hallucinations alone. Instead, their presence serves to confirm impressions received from a complex clinical picture that can include withdrawal and social isolation, impairment of role functioning, bizarre dress or actions, inappropriate or blunted affect, or "markedly peculiar" behavior.

In cultures such as that of Puerto Rico, it is difficult to distinguish between psychotic expressions—hallucinations and delusions—and visions and experiences of spirits, because the latter are a very real part of the culturally constituted environment of many people. Particularly in cases like Celia's, where persecutory voices were not present (or at least not reported) and where (as will later be described) the healing efforts of the Spiritists were successful, we might even question the validity of the concepts behind the definitions of hallucinations and delusions. Singer (1976) raises an interesting point when he notes that people less oriented toward fantasizing and daydreaming are more likely to become aware of their inner thoughts when severely disturbed and attribute them to external sources. As described in Chapter 3, the conversion experiences of Spiritist healers also include the attribution of certain internal experiences to external spirit beings. However, this attribution is made by someone other than the experiencer.

From the psychological viewpoint, the images of Spiritist believers are extremely elaborate but so also are those of some schizophrenics, especially with regard to social roles and interactions. Although they *appear* to be similar, there is one great difference: Visions and experiences of spirits are all framed by real and complex relationships—between medium-healers and their clients, between healers and spirits, and between clients and spirits. In contrast, the schizophrenic person usually withdraws from social interaction, and his imaginings are typically aspects of an internal dialogue. Moreover, as Singer notes (1976), the schizophrenic individual, when in a psychotic state, seems to lack the ability to communicate his visions and images.

Spiritist visions, on the other hand, although possessing a large variety of detail, actually conform to rather narrowly defined patterns. For example, animals are definitely not spirits, even though a spirit might form (*plasmar*) the vision of an animal in an individual as a metaphor for a human situation. This is fairly rare. But Spiritists do distinguish between visions and what they call "mental confusion." When the content of a vision does not conform to expected patterns, it is rejected as a "true" experience of spirits. The case of Juana, discussed at a case review session by both Spiritists and therapists, illustrates these distinctions.

Juana

Juana, twenty-seven years old and unmarried, was described by a Spiritist as a client whose problems

> began with malaise, crying, and always saying there was a "serpent at the door of the kitchen" in her home. She said that "the serpent changed into different shapes," and she became so emotional that her mother became very sad and came to me for help. At the *centro* Juana would not approach the table, saying that there was "a serpent on it who would harm" her. The healer's response

> was to tell Juana that there was no serpent, whereupon Juana backed away and fell into a fit of prolonged crying. Assistants then prepared a *bálsamo* (energy-charged water) which they flicked upon the young woman. She slowly stopped crying, took her hands from her face, and cried, "Oh, my God, thank God!" Juana then calmed down and was receptive to the healer.

We were told that for over two years this medium visited Juana at her home and "gave her passes" until she seemed to forget both the snake and her fears. However, her father and uncle repeated their drunken performance of knocking at her bedroom door late one night, and Juana again saw the serpent. Because the healer was on a trip to the United States, Juana's mother took her to the crisis division of a mental health center where she began to take off her clothes and scream. She was then hospitalized at a private psychiatric hospital. However, her mother became frightened when her daughter lost twenty-five pounds within a few weeks and secured a pass for her when the medium returned. The healer again worked with Juana, even keeping her at her home for weekends or weeks at a time. After six months, Juana was discharged from the hospital and did not return; but she did remain on antipsychotic medication. When she fell into another crisis, she was taken instead to the Spiritist healer. After approximately eleven years, Juana no longer had psychotic episodes but did become diabetic. The healer accounted for this change by saying that her "mind became better." Juana never married but left home to live with a niece. She was currently caring for her niece's children and was much calmer. The healer noted that Juana improved when she did not have to live with her father.

During the case discussion, Juana was never identified as "in development." Rather, the healer who treated her said "her mind had been very affected" and that she had "suffered a nervous shock," "an emotion so great that she saw the serpent." We reflected upon this as an example of Spiritist healers' recognition that people like Juana are emotionally disturbed to a far greater extent than most of their clients. People who are less disturbed but have visions are said to be developing their mediumistic faculties. However, although Juana was not diagnosed as "in development," her condition was still attributed to spirits who responded to and mirrored her difficulties with family members. There was also an allusion to hereditary factors predisposing Juana to a condition of "craziness," but this idea was not advanced as an explanation for the cause of her illness.

Comments from project participants with regard to the dream about an iguana (see Chapter 4) illustrate that Spiritists make a vague distinction between "abnormal" and acceptable visionary content. They were somewhat divided as to the identity of the iguana. One healer thought that it represented a very backward spirit, but another emphatically declared that spirits cannot be animals. The second Spiritist healer supported the latter opinion by making the observation that the spirit's "origin is divine because it comes directly from the Creator-Father." These different opinions were more or less resolved by a third healer, who said: "A spirit cannot convert itself into an animal. It is the effect of the imaginative aspect of a person that promotes a mental disturbance; because of this she sees an animal instead of a person. Seeing animals are imaginative errors." Thus it appeared clear that both Juana's vision of a serpent and Celia's strange ideas about her pregnant state are viewed by the Spiritists as the result of "mental confusion" brought about by situational, hereditary, and familial circumstances, all reflected in and echoed by spirit invasions. But animal visions are not considered to be true experiences of spirits, who are always anthropomorphic in appearance, because spirits *are* people as Spiritists define them.

Further Thoughts on Hallucinations and Visions

If reported sensations and visions of spirits are not signs of psychiatric illness, then what are they in psychological terms? When they are part of an initiatory experience, I have viewed them (in Chapter 3) as healthy and complementary adjuncts to changes in core self-identity and a new awareness of a part-self, a personal attribute to be used in the service of healing oneself and others. But when they are identified by Spiritists in some people who resist "development" as mediums or in those whom mediums do not view as "in development," how can they be interpreted from the perspective of clinical psychiatry or psychodynamic theory?

Westermeyer's interpretation (1987a, 1987b:10) is that "Hallucinations and preternatural experiences may also be difficult to separate. This is especially true when the patient's group values such experiences as trance, communicating with spirits or gods, vision quests and so forth." He suggests that such experiences have six characteristics that make them diametrically opposite to hallucinations: (1) the community and family usually support the experience, (2) the experience is time limited (and, I might add, expected to be), (3) the behavior prior to the experience and afterward is socially appropriate and productive, (4) the experiencer gains in social esteem and prestige, (5) there are no psychopathological signs or symptoms, and (6) the experience is culturally congruent (or patterned in a particular, expectable way, as I have discussed previously). Although I have alluded to all of the above characteristics in prior chapters, here I must emphasize that what is considered "psychopathological" is a judgment tailored by a particular medical or healing system. For Puerto Ricans who are not doctors and think in popular rather than medical terms, the judgment of whether a vision is not "normal and expectable" is in part based on an assessment of whether the individual is thought to suffer from or "have madness." Spiritists, on the other hand, generally view all preternatural experiences as visions of spirits. However, they say that some visions and auditory and other unusual sensations are not expectable types of experience but are the result of illness that affects the nervous system, which in turn causes "mental confusion" and aberrant experiences of spirits.

In psychodynamic theory, relatively few ideas have been advanced of ways to distinguish hallucinations from visionary experiences. Williams (1965:42) long ago offered an interesting perspective that allows for the cultural patterning of preternatural experiences and the consideration that visions can be aberrant and dysfunctional even when a community approves of them. He suggested that "it seems much more rational to attempt to discriminate between nonschizophrenic hallucinatory phenomena on the basis of the symbolic meaning they have for people experiencing them. That is, if one can interact with a hallucinated figure meaningfully [and adaptively, one might add] and attain gratification from it, this would only serve to strengthen one's psychic economy." Williams studied patients who were nineteen to twenty-two years of age in a reformatory setting, whom he described as "narcissistic." They had previously been diagnosed as "schizophrenic reaction, paranoid type." All of these young men longed to be dependent upon someone they viewed as benevolent; when they didn't have an actual relationship of this type, they constructed one—in "fantasy." Based on this experience, Williams distinguished between the meaning of their visions (which he labeled "hallucinations") and those of schizophrenics in that the relationship with the imagined person was not one of "clinging dependency" but instead a "more nearly symbiotic relationship." Not only were these men confined and deprived of opportunities for satifactory relationships but they also were incapable of trusting a real person in order to realize the kind of relationship they needed and desired. They therefore envisioned dead relatives as their imagined "magic helpers," just as do many Spiritists when they first begin to "develop" their faculties.

In the case of the adolescent girl described next, what was diagnosed as an acute psychotic episode was accompanied (or perhaps caused) by her change in feelings about a spirit-vision that had reoccurred over six years. As we noted, the Spiritists reviewing this case in response to a presentation by the psychologist treating the girl saw her visions as a sign of spiritual development.

Blanca Rosa

> Fourteen years old and in the fifth grade, Blanca Rosa had a history of school problems. While at school one day, she suffered from severe *ataques de llanto* (crying spells) and shouting, which had never before occurred. When brought to the mental health center two days later, she related that she saw her dead sister every night beside her bed. This sister died suddenly of a brain tumor at sixteen years of age; Blanca Rosa was then only eight years old. They had been

> especially close in this large family of ten children; Blanca's sister had read to her, helped with her school assignments, and slept with her.
>
> Blanca said that prior to her crisis at school, the vision of her sister had been a comforting one; but now it was telling her to run away from their father because he was "Satan" and would harm her. Blanca's father is also in treatment at the mental health center, having been an alcoholic who physically abused his wife and children. In the past he had singled out the older sister [the oldest of his children] on whom to vent his anger when he came home after a binge. He had struck her on the head many times. Blanca Rosa said that she believed her father had killed her sister even though he was no longer abusive to his family and had stopped drinking.

The psychologist told the group that she thought that much of the problem lay in the fact that the family had not observed any of the death rituals, such as the rosaries, the viewing, or the funeral mass. This girl's death became a hidden event, and they never visited her grave. She accounted for the fact that Blanca Rosa had become upset by the vision of her sister, after it had provided comfort for over six years, by suggesting a newly emerged defense mechanism now influencing Blanca's assessment of her father; she had begun to "project hostility" toward him. The therapist's interpretation included reference to the nature of adolescence as a developmental stage in which young people resent and reject their parents, in order to account for Blanca's change of perception of her father.

In response to this presentation, the Spiritists offered their interpretation of the vision, one that emphasized their concern that the emotional valence of the vision had changed. As mentioned earlier, a deceased female relative often appears as the first spirit protector-guide, and this was the Spiritists' explanation of why the sister appeared to Blanca. And, also as usual, it was felt by all of the Spiritist healers that the spirit of the dead sister was putting her agony into her younger sister and scaring her into certain realizations about their father, reinforcing a deep-seated fear of him. (In fact, Blanca had indicated that her father's behavior seemed quite distant emotionally. He interacted very little with her.) The healers also implied that there was the possibility that his sexual interest had surfaced now that Blanca Rosa was entering puberty. They saw the sister's spirit as positive and beneficial, even if it aroused fear in Blanca Rosa, because the spirit was "her mother in a former life." And Blanca Rosa was seen by the Spiritists as extremely isolated emotionally. They "saw" that her mother was passive and preoccupied with her other children and her difficult husband. What Blanca Rosa needed, according to the healers, was someone who would become a close friend and listen to her talk about her fears and distress. The sister's spirit must be instructed to be aware of the distress she is causing Blanca so that she can once again be a source of support for Blanca Rosa. This is the same "socialization" process to which all potential spirit guides are subjected.

Treatment and Outcome of Schizophrenia

By examining the largest sample of cases, it was possible to assess the frequency of various treatments that mental health workers prescribed for schizophrenic patients. Antipsychotic and other medications were the treatments used with greatest frequency. Some of the common drugs used were Mellaril (thioridazine), 51 percent; Tranxene (clorazepate dipotassium), 23 percent; Prolixin (fluphenazine hydrochloride), 14 percent; and Thorazine (chlorpromazine), 12 percent. Elavil (amitriptyline) was used in about 10 percent of the cases. In 34 percent of the cases the type of drug was not specified. Other types of therapies included "supportive therapy" (38 percent) and individual therapy (51 percent). Apart from occasional marital therapy and other special modalities, drug treatment seemed to be the most frequent choice, assisted by a day treatment program for a period of two weeks to several months—especially when the patient's family was burdened by her (or his) care. Hospitalization was a last resort for frustrated families who still carried the main burden of chronically mentally ill people, just as they had some twenty-five years ago (Rogler and Hollingshead, 1965). This reflects the norm in Puerto Rico—that unmarried people (especially women) live with their natal families, particularly those who are handicapped in any way.

Because there were so few Spiritist cases reclassified in the schizophrenia category, the frequencies of various treatments cannot be assessed. However, in a number of cases and case discussions, Spiritists referred to certain clients as "spiritually crazy," and mediums also commented on the psychotherapeutic treatment of diagnosed schizophrenics in the case review sessions. As mentioned earlier, chronically ill people are often followed for many years by Spiritist healers, who not only treat them at the *centros* but also see them in their homes during periods of crisis. In the case of Celia, who was seen both at a Spiritist *centro* and at the community mental health center, the Spiritist healer who treated her said that only one *causa* spirit was "passed" on her behalf. That spirit said that the client and her mother needed a great deal of "spiritual help," and they should continue to attend sessions as often as possible. Other then this one occasion, Celia was only given "magnetic passes" because the medium working with her believed that "passing her *causas*" would worsen her condition. The reason given for this was that Celia's spirit was outside of her body, and therefore the *causa* spirit could take it over much more easily. The medium explained that "this is especially the case when clients are on medication, *endrogada* [that is, drugged up on an antipsychotic or other medication] due to the great intoxication of the medication. I have to know who she really is, and I can never know this while she is drugged."

This echoed what we had heard many times; Spiritist healers have a very negative attitude toward clients' taking antipsychotic medication. Many say that such medication "clouds the mind." Thus they frequently come into direct conflict with psychiatric mandates for pharmacological treatment. We had to note that their disapproval of antipsychotic medication was steadfastly held, even when the Spiritist healers became aware (through the Therapist-Spiritist Project) of the important role of medication in the treatment of psychotic patients and despite their positive views on most other types of medication. We discussed the idea that the Spiritists' attitudes toward antipsychotic medications is one of a predominant value that guides their practice. They preach that a client must be accepted just as she is, and no one should be put off by strange behavior. For example, although the medium who worked with Celia viewed her problems as stemming from a high state of "mental confusion in which she lacks values," the medium also said that Celia's behavior was due to impetuosity, and she had no idea of goals to guide her actions. Moreover, her mother did not want her to become oriented to life and thus "tied" her daughter to her.

Because Celia was the focus of an experimental coordination of treatment between a mental health worker and a Spiritist healer, an agreement was reached for medication to be withdrawn. Celia showed great improvement a few weeks later after she had attended day treatment full-time for one month (subsequently, three times per week for four months), had seen her therapist once per week, and had made biweekly visits to the *centro*. Given the variety of treatments, it is impossible to say which or what was responsible for her improvement, although she appeared to the Project team to be free of psychotic symptoms, such as hearing voices, delusions, and confused thought processes. This seemed to be a very exceptional recovery; however, we were aware that approximately 40 percent of people diagnosed as schizophrenic, especially those with early onset of the illness, experience remission of symptoms for long periods and about 20 percent seem to recover completely (Lehmann and Cancro, 1985). Celia's improvement could have been due to spontaneous remission or to the increased levels of attention she was receiving, regardless of the specific type of treatment. (Or it is even possible that she was not suffering from schizophrenia at all, although she had been rediagnosed by the CMHC psychiatrist and two psychologists from the Project who interviewed her.) Celia steadily improved for over a year and then began to skip sessions in both the CMHC and the *centro*, until she failed altogether to come in for treatment. At one point her therapist noted that Celia had an episode after each failed love affair. And so, as predicted, after about fifteen months Celia became involved with another man and went to live with his family. Shortly afterward she suffered another brief episode and took an overdose of medication. Just a week or so later, she went to her mother's home saying she wanted to return there to live. We followed her for about a year and a half before losing track of her. But about five years later, one of the Spiritists told us that Celia had returned to the *centro* and seemed to be doing well.

Rogler and Hollingshead (1965) report on how the Spiritist *centro* supports the schizophrenic (and his family) by offering him or her "an alternative role that encompasses and sanctions his idiosyncratic symptoms, and, moreover, one that does not impose on him the burden of stigma." Although this is partly true for some schizophrenic patients I observed, it is rare that they are groomed to work as mediums. I knew of two well-known healer-mediums who had each suffered more than one psychotic episode and had been hospitalized. Their illnesses were obviously in remission, and they were symptom-free when they worked the spirits at that time. One woman was regarded as especially effective with psychotic, mentally retarded, and chronically ill clients. But there were many other participants at *centro* sessions who, although diagnosed as mentally ill, held no special status.

We reflected upon the idea that the successes reported by Spiritist healers with people who suffered psychotic episodes seem more readily explained by the high degree of tolerance they have toward bizarre behavior, especially behavior psychiatry would label as delusional. Another factor is the concentrated attention and caring attitude that some healers give to chronically mentally ill people, as illustrated in the cases of both Juana and Celia. In addition, and perhaps most important, symptoms of schizophrenia acquire meaningfulness in the context of Spiritist beliefs, in direct contrast to their being considered abnormal and unwanted by mental health professionals. In this way, the ill person's self-esteem is not damaged by Spiritist treatment and can even be experienced as being enhanced. In fact, people with schizophrenia, when not in a psychotic episode, are not seen as abnormal. For example, the Spiritist healer who treated Celia stated rather emphatically: "She is not crazy. It's [really] a moral dilemma. She could be a prostitute, but she becomes so upset after an affair that she retreats from it through her [bizarre] behavior."

Here I want to note that some of the Spiritists' attitudes toward psychiatric treatment did change as a result of the Project. But at a *centro* session we attended early in the Project when we were recruiting participants, their attitudes were evident in the message given one client. She was told, "I want you to cathart, speak, be tranquil, a new person with desire to work and triumph. The Beloved One will help. We don't need psychiatrists. The spirits here are the psychiatrists of the universe."

We observed that there is a basic tendency in Spiritism, expressed in many ways, to focus on the strain toward normality, defined as ideal moral behavior, rather than on the absence of mental illness. We discussed Warner's view (1976–1977) that Western psychiatric discourse on mental illness represents a static view of mental illness. The use of nouns to describe patients—for example, "She is a schizophrenic" or "She is bipolar"—imparts the idea that the disease is an entity rather than a process that can change in far-reaching ways. Psychiatric diagnoses then become inseparable from the people who have been labeled, which leads to their feeling degraded and lends itself to further denigration. The Spiritist approach to all illness as conditions visited upon the afflicted avoids this concretization and the resultant negative identity that is augmented by or develops with mental illness. The concept of chronicity has no place in the Spiritist scheme of things; illness and severe problems, viewed as processes of spirit intervention in one's current life, inevitably change—even if it takes more than one lifetime. The strength of this approach for the ill person is the possibility of cautious hopefulness. (See also Koss, 1987).

As we pursued the Project over the years, we had to acknowledge that Spiritism does not systematically provide as complete a range of treatments for severely disordered people as do community mental health center programs with partial hospitalization, day care, and outpatient services. However, as was observed long ago by Rogler and Hollingshead (1965), the *centros* support people with long-term mental illness within their community setting. Garrison (1978), in an ingeniuous study in the New York Puerto Rican community, compared the "naturally occurring support systems" of a neighborhood sample of nonschizophrenic women with a matched sample of women diagnosed with schizophrenias in both inpatient and hospital care. As has been found for schizophrenic women in other populations, these ill women generally relied only on one best friend. They were overdependent upon a medical institution, commonly had fewer kin and nonkin in their social networks, and were overdependent on one or a few family members from another generation. However, contrary to expectations created by studies of schizophrenics in other U.S. communities, there was relatively little difference between their relationships with nonkin and those of the nonschizophrenic women. That is, a majority of the schizophrenic women were church-goers, knew their neighbors, and reported other friendships. In other words, they were not particularly isolated or withdrawn from social contacts. All had some history of involvement with Spiritism, and most relied on a healing cult as a primary source of help. This is the same pattern we found in Puerto Rico, illustrated by the cases we have described in this chapter.

Many recent studies show that community support, in addition to regular medication, protects the diagnosed schizophrenic from frequent relapses. The most severe and chronic patients in the current sample, such as Herminia, had early suffered complete abandonment by family members and were unable to maintain a conjugal relationship. However, even severely disturbed women have had opportunities to marry or live consensually, which perhaps speaks to greater tolerance toward symptoms of psychosis among the less-educated and nonmedical members of Latin societies.

We found it interesting that Spiritist responses to diagnosed schizophrenics follow the guidelines set out by newer psychoeducational methods for their families (Falloon et al., 1981). These specify that criticism, overinvolvement, and intensity in interactions with a person suffering from schizophrenia will hasten relapse. We observed that the mediums seemed to intuitively understand this, as illustrated by the stated inhibition on "passing" the *causa* spirits affecting Celia and by the uncritical maternal warmth provided over many years to Juana whenever she experienced distress generated by family relationships. In addition, mediums are also intuitively aware of the need for social support. In the case review session where Blanca Rosa was discussed, they vividly imaged her situation by "seeing" her in a "box with cement walls." She was described as suffering because she had no friends and because her mother gave her too little attention. In fact, they suggested that her therapist become her "friend" and teacher.

Observations and Thoughts

Although the mandate of the Community Mental Health Program in Puerto Rico is to provide crisis intervention and supportive care for chronically mentally ill people, Spiritist practices are an important adjunct to community care. Spiritists' healing work with people suffering schizophrenic illnesses appears to be a significant factor in lessening the need for hospitalization for many women diagnosed as schizophrenic. Largely through the concentrated attention some healers provide to the ill person and their assistance to frustrated family members, fewer people suffering severe mental illness may relapse. (However, it would require a double-blind study to demonstrate the effect of Spiritist practices on relapse.) It also seems likely that Spiritists help some people who have not presented to a psychiatric clinic but who are suffering from cognitive and behavioral disorders that might be diagnosed as schizophrenic. In our samples, we found three cases where this was a possibility. However, because our method was based on comparison of complaint profiles and Spiritists do not classify visionary experiences as hallucinatory or delusional (and also fail to note cognitive dysfunctions such as "loose associations"), such comparisons are unlikely to point to undiagnosed cases of schizophrenia. Moreover, the idiom of "having nerves" as a popular way to refer to psychosis masks a condition that might be diagnosed as schizophrenia but does not get presented to a clinic unless the afflicted person becomes burdensome to her family.

We found one pattern common to families of schizophrenic women in Puerto Rico of special interest. If we agree with Al-Issa (1982) that schizophrenic women who behave angrily and assertively are using role reversal as an expression of rebellion against societal norms of passivity and compliance, we might speculate that this is associated with a particular family pattern. In this type of family environment, there is an emotionally distant, often abusive but feared father and an ineffectual, passive but caring mother, inadequate to the task of protecting her daughter from hurt (or sexual abuse) inflicted by the father. As in the cases of Celia and Juana, the daughter's anger is then directed at the mother's failure to nurture and protect. We might ask why the father is not more of a target for the ill woman's hostility? To speculate, it seems that many women as daughters have low expectations of their fathers, but their expectations of their mothers are quite high. A kind of psychological splitting occurs that produces "bad" mothers and "good" (or uninvolved but well-intentioned) fathers, who are not targeted for anger by daughters, even in highly dysfunctional families.

We were aware that psychiatry clearly recognizes that stressful life events may push a person at risk for mental illness into a psychotic episode, which can become a chronic disorder. Both therapists and Spiritists agree in principle that people with bizarre behavior and affect need supportive relationships to keep relapse at bay. Each type of healer assists with this aspect of treatment within the institutional framework in which she works. When Spiritists, for example, take an interest in a person afflicted by schizophrenia, they are able to provide psychological shelter and protection within the community, thus avoiding the sometimes negative effects of hospitalization. Mental health professionals, on the other hand, work to free the ill person from her most damaging symptoms as soon as possible. They use antipsychotic medication and a variety of partial hospitalization programs aimed at resocializing the patient into more adaptive life skills and behavior. It is of considerable interest that despite very different conceptualizations about the etiology of schizophrenia and the meaning of the complaints presented by these patients, the general outcomes of treatment for acute episodes by mental health professionals and Spiritist healers can be quite similar.[2]

Notes

1. See also Gaviria and Wintrob, 1976, who report on belief in and use of Spiritist practices among psychiatric patients in two communities in the state of Connecticut.

2. See Koss, 1987, for a study of self-reported outcomes of the two types of treatment. This study, however, examined individual complaints, not diagnostic categories.

9

Nerves and Anxiety Disorders

Nerves are almost always physical.

—An *Espiritista*, 1987

To say that there are many reasons why women in Puerto Rico are anxious is only to repeat the dreary litany of their marital and family problems, as well as their deep feelings of abandonment and the fear that they cannot survive alone. As described earlier, both men and women find Puerto Rico a difficult society to negotiate. Women find their lives especially full of problems because they so often lack a sense of personal power. Surprisingly, many middle-class women negate the potential social power they acquire, through good salaries or prestige gained in professional life, in favor of the power of significant male others. Their spouses or partners much more often feel empowered to make decisions that can disregard these women's achievements. The women in these chapters, who are patients or clients, come largely from poorer social groups, which lack education as well as opportunities to acquire personal power in whatever form. Their feelings of hopelessness over a personal future are often realistic appraisals of the difficulties of trying to support themselves and their children without a partner's help. This unhappy realism exacerbates attitudes of dependence associated with being a woman and even seems to arouse a fear of independence.

Given the indeterminacy of Puerto Rico's political status and economic direction and the continuing onslaught of cultural, social, and economic changes that typify its social life, there is a general feeling of uncertainty and considerable concern about future plans or dreams. Family dysfunction is a toxic additive to an already potent brew of doubts and fears for the future. Distress over family problems (such as teenage rebellion and substance abuse or a husband's alcoholic abusiveness) adds to with the stress that poor, uneducated women already feel as a result of their predisposition to personal indeterminacy.[1] The effect (and affect) of this dual source of stress (inner and outer as well as multidimensional) is vividly illustrated by one of the Spiritist healers, Evangelina, who without prompting described herself as a "very nervous person," "very tense physically," and sometimes so "dizzy" that she "cannot walk." Possessed of a very sensitive, intelligent nature but only a fifth grade education, she worked for years at routine and often menial jobs in a tobacco factory. Evangelina reports that she suffered a series of *ataques* during this period. But one day something snapped, and she felt she could "never again roll another cigar," whatever happened. She suffered a prolonged illness, which she describes as having been initiated by a crisis, an "*ataque de nervios*," in which she felt her body weaken and suffered a "mental block." Evangelina succumbed to the crisis for almost two years and was left without income or family members who cared about her. A childhood friend took care of her; she also began to develop as a medium.

When we (and two other Project participants, a psychiatrist and a psychologist) viewed Evangelina from a psychiatric perspective, through the lens of the Diagnostic and Statistical Manual (APA, 1987), we thought that she suffered from "agoraphobia," initiated by "panic attacks." She herself describes her condition as chronic "nervousness," which keeps her from leaving the house except on special occasions.

Because she became a lecturer and presenter at a number of Project events (after being recruited as a participant), the narration of Evangelina's story was intertwined with Project situations. Much of it is recounted later in this chapter. It is of special interest because she so well illustrates how one individual can simultaneously incorporate both patient and healer characteristics. "Nervios" (or *nerviosidad*, "nervousness"), the idiom of distress that she frequently uses, is a very popular expression that can identify severe anxiety but is also at the center of a network of related complaints that incorporate references to somatic distress as well as interpersonal problems. The two English terms, "nervousness" and "anxiety," are not equivalent as descriptions of experience of emotional distress. "Anxiety" as "intensive apprehension, fearfulness, or terror associated with feelings of impending doom" (APA, 1987) implies a distressful inner state or emotion that if severe can manifest in disordered behavior, causing distress to both sufferer and others. In contrast, "*nervios*" (as "nervousness") simultaneously involves body structure, a chaotic emotional state, many somatic complaints, and, particularly, a sense of loss of control over one's perceptions, behavior, and surroundings. As will be illustrated later, these idioms also connote feelings of bad treatment or rejection at the hands of family members, together with a sense of combined physical and social instability. (See also Guarnaccia et al., 1989, and Guarnaccia and Farias, 1988.)

This chapter will explore the meanings "nervousness" has for women who complain of it, an idiom of distress encapsulated within a network of meanings that refer to stressful life events, inherent personal attributes, and predispositions to emotional distress. We will also explore the relationship of the "nerves" complex to the partially overlapping psychiatric classification "anxiety disorders." As in the last two chapters, I include descriptions of the ways each type of healer explains and diagnoses, locates the cause, and develops strategies to treat emotional distress described either as severe anxiety or as a permutation of the condition of "nervousness."

The Nature of Nervousness, Intranquility, and *Ataques de Nervios*

"Nerves" (and "*nervios*") as a "culturebound symptom" or popular complaint has been widely documented in societies in North, Central, and South America (Low, 1981, 1985; Guarnaccia and Farias, 1988; Davis and Whitten, 1988; Davis and Guarnaccia, 1989; Garrison, 1977b). It was first formalized by medical notions advanced by famous early physicians—Hippocrates (ca. 5th to 4th centuries BC) and especially Galen (2nd century AD)—who thought that "nerves" were the physical structures that communicated between body and mind (Davis and Whitten, 1988). Later medical traditions in eighteenth- and nineteenth-century America and Europe focused on the physical properties of nerves and how they caused or contributed to both somatic and psychiatric conditions—infertility, on the one hand, madness and mania on the other. Environmental conditions as well as moral turpitude were at various times held responsible for "bad nerves." By the end of the nineteenth century, nerves inevitably became linked with emotions and were viewed as causing most emotional disorders. "Nerves" were held accountable for a myriad of symptoms, moods, physical sensations, and behavioral disturbances. (See Davis and Whitten, 1988, for a fuller history of "nerves.")

Perhaps through the popularization of early medical notions, translated from sixteenth- and seventeenth-century Spanish medicine, "nervousness" has become a general label for disordered emotions and behavior in Puerto Rico, as elsewhere. Without necessarily being associated with serious or chronic conditions of illness, "nerves" basically refer to temperament and to emotions that disturb and prevent "tranquility." However, compared to other societies, such as Costa Rica, the pattern of meanings connoted by the term "nerves" in Puerto Rico and the particular conditions it refers to (or accounts for) have some unique features.

Counted together, "intranquility," "nerves," and "nervousness" vie with sleep disturbances as the most frequent types of complaints presented to all of the healers and health professionals and are frequent complaints in all of the eight diagnostic categories. However, we noted that a few complaints, such as "*ansiedad*," "*agitamiento*" (agitation), and "*desasociego*" (restlessness), were fairly frequently associated with "nerves" in the profile associated with the nerves/anxiety disorders category (see Appendix, Table 1.A). We observed that participants often made a distinction between "intranquility" as situational and commonly connoting a *state* of apprehension and fear and "nervousness" as a *trait* or expected reaction of people suffering from disturbed "nerves." Because of this difference, "intranquility" as a complaint was assessed separately in the complaint profiles associated with each diagnostic category as well as considered separately in my descriptions of patients' and clients' experiences of anxiety, nervousness, and other similar distressful feelings.

Some researchers have described *nervios* as a popular term for an illness state (Garrison, 1977b), such as when Puerto Ricans say they "suffer from nerves" (*padecer de los nervios*) or are "sick from nerves" (*enferma de los nervios*). When referred to in these ways, a mental disorder is not necessarily denoted. Moreover, "nerves" or "nervousness" are frequent complaints that patients used when presenting almost any type of physical distress. The expressions we recorded that are popularly used to describe a person who would be (or was) diagnosed as chronically mentally ill by a mental health professional are slightly different, as discussed earlier in Chapter 8. In these expressions about "nerves," there is more of a sense of an inherent disability passed on through family lines. We noted the difficulty (even popularly) of the task of distinguishing "craziness" from normality, because "nervousness" as experience and popular complaint is so widespread. We reflected upon the notion that this was a purposeful social deception to mask the stigma of "*locura*." Moreover, when we looked at "nerves" in the context of the nerves/anxiety disorders category of emotional distress, the confusion is compounded because people who "suffer from nerves" are much more likely to have a sudden *ataque de nervios*. Some patients, clients, and healers said that the inner heat commonly felt by the sufferer builds and can be set off by an event or series of happenings perceived as stressful. We observed that women (and some men) succumbed to an episode of loss of consciousness initiated by sudden screams that were followed by falling flat upon the ground, twitching, flailing, and moaning. Such extreme behavior was accepted and even expected as a manifestation of extreme grief in women at a velorio (wake) or funeral of a close relative. I have sometimes seen *ataques* at viewings where the woman is supported by her relatives, given something pungent to smell, and sometimes held or held down to keep from hurting herself. On one such occasion, a distant male cousin of the deceased flung himself prone onto the floor in an *ataque*. Whispered comments indicated that many felt this was not appropriate, because his grief should not have overwhelmed him.

The phenomenon of *ataques de nervios* in Puerto Rico has been interpreted in the literature by a number of observers. It was labeled the "Puerto Rican Syndrome" by Rubio et al. (1955). (See also Mehlman, 1961; Fernández Marina, 1961; Garrison, 1979; and Guarnaccia et al., 1989a, 1989b.) Pursuing this literature, the reader might ask, as we did, why so many differing psychodynamic interpretations and psychiatric labels have been applied to this phenomenon. Psychiatrists early noted that *ataques* among male army recruits were associated with many different types of mental disorder, ranging from schizophrenia to acute states of conversion. They felt that calling it a "syndrome" masked an understanding of the "real disease process" (Mehlman, 1961). However, other observers of *ataques* in psychiatric and other settings have viewed them as a hysterical, dissociative phenomena (Fernández Marina, 1961; Garrison, 1977b). There is some agreement among the authors that *ataques* represent the "discharge of repressed or suppressed anger" (Garrison, 1977b:439) and that Puerto Ricans lack sufficient opportunities for discharging anxiety or aggressive impulses (Rothenberg, 1964).[2] Most writers also agree that *ataques* are closely related to familial conflict and occur at times of extreme personal stress, such as after accidents that befall oneself or a loved one. In my opinion, lumping together cases of men and women when exploring the phenomenon of *ataques* obscures answers to the question of what *ataques* mean to those who experience them. According to many observations, the ways men and women relate to and express anger are very different.

The case narratives presented in this chapter are of three types: (1) cases of anxiety disorder presented to mental health professionals, (2) cases in which the complaints of "nervousness" and "intranquility" are presented to Spiritist healers (whether or not the complaints meet criteria for "anxiety disorders"), and (3) organic problems presented to doctors in which women complain of "nervousness." Through an analysis of narratives about illness and emotional disorder, I attempt to fathom the meanings of "nervousness" as (1) an expected aspect of the experience of distress in many women, (2) a popular illness category, (3) a metaphoric way of connoting interpersonal layers of experience of strain associated with interpersonal difficulties, and (4) a condition that can erupt into acute episodes of dissociative experience (*ataques de nervios* and other *ataques*) in a few, chronically nervous women. As in previous chapters, I also explore how we interpreted "nervousness" as a complaint, as well as an experience, to be related to the psychiatric diagnosis of anxiety disorder.

Gender, Nervousness, and Anxiety Disorders

We often reflected on the questions: Are *nervios* more frequent in women than in men? Do women suffer more from emotional distress than do men? Or do women perceive their lives to be more stressful and more commonly express this in terms of "nerves?" The category of complaints called "nerves" in this study included the complaints of "nervousness," "intranquility," "anxiety," "restlessness," "agitation," and "whiplashes [*látigos*] in the nerves." "Nerves" was presented to therapists (doctors and mental health workers) by 31 percent (245 cases) of all the women as clients and patients over all categories in the largest sample and to Spiritist healers by 28 percent of their women clients (63 cases). Similarly, the complaint of "nerves" was presented to their therapists by 33 percent (218 cases) of male patients and to Spiritists by 30 percent (35 cases) of male clients. We must conclude that men who present their distress to therapists, doctors, or Spiritists manifest "nerves" as often as women do. However, it should also be noted that men present themselves less frequently to these health care givers. Because my data are not derived from strictly randomized samples, frequencies cannot be compared with a high degree of confidence. With this caution in mind, we can note that in the largest sample of the three on which this study is based, composed of 1,769 cases, women are overrepresented as patients by approximately 28 percent and as Spiritist clients by approximately 50 percent, assuming that both men and women had equal opportunities to seek help from these providers.

When we looked at our data on people labeled by mental health professionals and doctors as suffering from anxiety disorders and who also presented the complaint of "nerves," there was almost no difference in frequency between men and women, even though there was a significant difference between men and women in the total number of cases diagnosed as "anxiety disorders" (79 males and 108 females). Sixty-three percent of the women diagnosed in the "anxiety disorder" category said they were "nervous" or suffered from "nerves." In contrast, 58 percent of the men diagnosed as having an anxiety disorder presented with "nervousness." An examination of both the careful epidemiological data presented by Canino and my own data shows that although women suffer more from some states labeled "anxiety disorder" (specifically, phobias), anxious men are almost equally as "nervous," according to self-reported complaints in clinical and Spiritist settings. Moreover, more than twice as many men diagnosed as having a physical rather than a mental illness presented as "nervous"; and more men (62 percent) than women (53 percent) diagnosed as "depressed" (dysthymic) said they were "nervous," even though women suffer dysthymia more than four times as often as do men in Puerto Rico. In cases of schizophrenia, the frequency was reversed: 55 percent of the women as compared to 38 percent of the men said they were "nervous." The commonness of this type of expression of distress, and its pattern in relation to psychiatric and physical illness among men and women, supports my interpretation of "nervousness" as something equivalent to a general notion of "stress" experienced as *in* the body. I will discuss cultural permutations on this popular concept and attend to its meaning as "stress" in the conclusion to this chapter.[3]

Cases of "Anxiety Disorders" and "Nerves"

A mental health technician presented the case of Clara, diagnosed as having an "anxiety reaction with depressive features" (DSMII, APA, 1968).

Clara reported that her "nerves went out of control" when her husband left her to go to the United States. We noted that the mental health worker did not identify Clara's episode as an "*ataque*," but it appeared to us to have been what now might be classified in psychiatry as a "minor panic attack." Clara responded to a tranquilizer and once-a-month psychotherapy sessions. She identified the cause of her distress as long-term problems in relationships with men and phobiclike fears associated with abandonment.

Clara

"My head hurts; I feel like I have a hole or emptiness; I am unable to sleep; my eyes are very irritated, and tears pour out." This was Clara's description of how she felt the day the doctor referred her to the mental health center. Her sleep was disturbed by "strange" dreams in which she was "lifted by her hair and sent to another world."

Thirty-five years of age with three daughters, Clara sheepishly says she is "separated." Her second husband left her only a few weeks ago. Her only income is from food stamps, since neither of her husbands send money "to feed their daughters." She maintains good relations with her siblings, who try to help her, but one brother is also being treated at the mental health center. When asked about her family, Clara says that she was "an orphan at four years of age. My father left our home and my mother raised us alone." Her second husband's departure appeared to be more than Clara could bear; it was this third major abandonment in her life that seemed to her and her therapist to precipitate her "nerves [going] out of control."

Clara reported she felt she had a "hole" or "vacuum" inside of her. We reflected upon our observation that this image was fairly common as a complaint symbolizing rejection and seemed to point to feelings of abandonment by a man whom Clara needed to sustain and protect her. Women look to men as "protectors" of their very survival, who contribute money but also keep the stresses of daily life from their thresholds. These feelings had long reigned in Clara's consciousness. The dissociative quality of Clara's dreams fits within the reported experience of an "*ataque de nervios*" as well as being a symptom of a "panic attack" in psychiatric diagnostic convention.

A description of another distressed woman's experience (recorded at a *centro* session where she sought help) shows how the Spiritists work with what mental health professionals would label "phobic anxiety." Delia's two main complaints ("seen" by the healers but confirmed by her) were "intranquility" and "nervousness," accompanied by "susto" (fear, fright) and "pain in one leg."

Delia

Four *videncias* are offered to Delia (a woman of thirty years) by three different mediums. First: "A spirit says that you are looking for a solution to material

> problems. You are involved in an accident, and your leg is in a cast." Second: "You are nervous and frightened. There is a chain that you are trying to disentangle. There is something that comes from another existence that has you entangled in the chain." Third: "There is a spirit in your spiritual tableau that wants you to have an accident." And fourth: "You are very naive. I am frank. It is a *guía* that possesses me. But you come with a spirit who has been watching you for a very long time. The spirit makes you restless. He interferes with everything. You have to pray, meditate. Keep coming [here], and maybe you can be helped. You have to have more faith."

After the session, we discussed the view that the suggestion to Delia was that she was fearful about accidents because she was "entangled" in an emotional morass brought on by a spirit. Moreover, her condition was "chronic" because the spirit had been around for a long time. This spirit evidence also contained the solution (treatment); that is, Delia should pray and meditate on spiritual matters instead of being preoccupied by "material" fears. The spirits implied that intranquility, anxiety, and fear can be countered, or at least controlled, by a spiritual attitude that would put her in touch with good spirits. The healers clearly distinguished Delia's feeling state as the problem and tended to take a preventative approach in light of what they perceived to be her vulnerability.

In Irene's story, presented by her therapist, a psychologist, we saw an example of extreme but sudden nervousness. From the perspective of current diagnostic fashion in psychiatry, we might label her episode of distress a "panic attack," but it would not meet the criteria for a panic disorder because it was not followed by at least two more attacks over a three-week period. (See also the discussion by Guarnaccia et al., 1989b).

Irene

> Irene is forty-three years old and not yet married. She returned to Puerto Rico for a vacation and told me she had had the following dream: "I was walking in a strange place in order to get home. I saw an iguana who became stuck to my left thigh. The iguana said, 'You are not going to find anyone to get you out of this.' I said, 'Yes, I will find someone.' I continued walking with the iguana stuck to me. I went into several houses and people laughed at me."
>
> Two days later Irene began to feel "a current in my neck, and my arm [the left one] felt like it was going to fall off." She also said she felt depressed and very anxious at times. She consulted several doctors and underwent tests for hearing, heart, and thyroid problems. Two weeks later she suffered her first "anxiety attack" when she reached into the oven to take out a cake. She had "palpitations," felt "intense fear that she would die," and began to "tremble" and "sweat." When she got to the doctor's office, he told her it was "emotional," an "anxiety attack," and prescribed a tranquilizer. Since that time she suffered

various attacks of anxiety. Irene said that she sought help because she was unable to "coordinate her thoughts and had almost no ability to concentrate."

We observed that, as reported by her therapist, Irene presented the events of her illness as if the dream had precipitated them; it certainly had shakened and frightened her. After probing for an event that might explain this first attack, the therapist reported that she could find nothing remarkable. Up until the time of the attack, Irene had led a single life as a secretary and interpreter and had taken on the responsibility of her mother and blind brother after her father left home. (He converted to the Pentecostal religion, and the family refused to follow him.) A sister and brother were married and lived away from home, but Irene had also helped to educate them. Despite her obvious devotion, she expressed feelings of "uselessness" with regard to helping her blind brother and mother. She had had a boyfriend some years ago who left the island and returned married; during the time of her vacation in Puerto Rico (when she had the dream), he took her to dinner and said that he was sorry he had not married her. She claimed not to care for him anymore and currently had another boyfriend whom she was planning to marry. But the therapist speculated that although Irene said she was content with her lot in life and reasonably happy, she was actually deeply hostile and resentful toward her brother and mother for limiting her opportunities to have her own life. She felt "stuck" in her obligation toward them.

We speculated whether the *ataques* offered Irene a way to be angry without having to *act* angrily. Abad and Boyce (1979:31) suggest that the *ataque* is a "culturally learned and sanctioned symptom precipitated by unsuccessfully repressed anger or sexual tension." This could mean that "nervousness" and "intranquility" symbolize "trapped anger." One-fourth of all the patients seen by mental health professionals in our project complained of "hostility" (that is, feeling "hostility," "anger," "hatred," or "desire to fight"). We thought that the complaint of anger or hostility might be a trade-off for another one-fourth who had "crying jags," because many women cry when they are unable to express anger. In Irene's case, both her therapist and our interviewer sensed that she exhibited a kind of bravado in the face of the burden of responsibilities she had carried for many years. Moreover, as one of the mental health professionals suggested, it may be almost impossible to direct anger at people (such as close family members) who have always given meaning to your life, because to do so would be tantamount to negating your own self-worth. In addition, Irene was considering whether she was able to continue working and so had found an indirect way to lighten the burden of her responsibilities toward her brother and mother by entering the sick role.

Various commentators on Irene's case suggested that rather than simply symbolizing "repressed anger," "nervousness" be interpreted as describing an effort to suppress one's assertiveness in situations where both inner personal values and outer social requirements collude in thwarting its expression. Irene told her therapist that her third priority, following decisions about whether to continue working and how to deal with her brother's problems, was to attend to "her own feelings."

On reviewing her treatment decisions, the therapist acknowledged that Irene was very desirous of "knowing herself" in order to "find something for herself." She therefore used Gestalt therapy as the main modality (Perls, 1951), having Irene work with her own subpersonalities (including the submerged angry part) and also taking on the roles of other people in order to explore how she had projected certain doubts and fears onto them. The therapist judged her approach to be quite successful and commented that the use of this therapeutic modality was possible because Irene was "more sophisticated" than most other patients.

The Spiritists' response to the presentation of this case was to approve of Gestalt as an appropriate therapeutic modality for Irene, pointing out that it seemed similar to working the spirits. However, the mediums then focused mainly on Irene's iguana dream. They argued about whether the iguana was actually a spirit or only a distorted picture of one. But they all seemed to agree that the dream contained transformational meaning; it signified that Irene's balance in life had been disrupted, and inner disorder had ensued—later to manifest as an *ataque*. The *ataque* was viewed by the healers as an eruption of feelings her psyche and body were no longer able to contain once inner harmony had been lost.

Clinic Findings

Fela

Fela, twenty-two years old, married with two children, presented at a primary care clinic with "headaches, insomnia, poor appetite, palpitations, anxiety, and anguish that she had suffered for seven months." The doctor (a Project participant) ordered a series of laboratory tests, all of which came back negative. While waiting for the results, she prescribed a tranquilizer and felt that she already knew that Fela's condition was "emotional." Her first encounter with Fela was described as difficult, because "she seemed very anxious, continually changing her position in the chair and wringing her hands." All vital signs seemed normal, including low blood pressure (systolic:110/diastolic:70) and a pulse rate of 68. She questioned Fela closely and got the following story.

> My husband is younger than I am and does not work. I work in a factory and pay my family's bills and care for my little sons [ages 1 and 3 years]. I leave them

> with a neighbor each morning, but sometimes I have to work overtime in order to earn enough money for our expenses; and I worry about them. Moreover, my husband brings me a series of problems. He drinks too much and stays out late at night. My mother died last year of breast cancer, and my father always demands my attention. Although I try to please him, it often seems impossible.

In discussing Fela's problems, both her doctor and the Spiritist healers at the case review session recognized that her job could be a potent stressor within the knot of problems she was experiencing. However, one medium pointed out that Fela's somatic complaints were an attempt to compel her husband to feel guilty and take on some of the burden. She commented: "Fela tries to use her illness to punish him. This is very characteristic of the Puerto Rican woman, to act like a martyr." Yet the mediums and the doctor also agreed that Fela's strong sense of responsibility toward her family actually kept her "from going crazy."

In reviewing hundreds of cases, we observed that "headaches" generally mean the distress is so severe that help must be sought; head pain commonly signals the need for health care and entrance into the sick role. It also indicates that the sufferer is overwhelmed with distressing circumstances perceived as beyond her control to change. These circumstances are usually interpersonal in nature; "head pain" often denotes feelings of disorientation with regard to significant others. Fela's distress seems to have been exacerbated by a feeling of lack of emotional support, especially from a mother who could be expected to be an unfailing source of empathy and emotional security. If she were diagnosed as having a psychiatric illness, it would probably be "generalized anxiety disorder," based upon criteria such as "anxious mood continuous for over a month," worry, fear, and anticipation of misfortune, as well as the physical sensations of palpitations and head pain (tension) (APA, 1987). Her insomnia and crying jags point to a depressive component in her distress, related to grief over the loss of her mother.

In other cases we recorded, young women (under forty) presented at a primary care facility with complaints of arthritis, hypertension, kidney infections, diabetes, and other illnesses, accompanied by "headaches" as well as "stomach pains" (the latter often described as "nerves in the stomach"). Although in our assessment their anxiety was not as debilitating as that experienced by those who meet criteria for an anxiety disorder, tranquilizers were frequently prescribed by doctors who reported that they identified their patients' conditions as partly due to "nerves." One woman complained that when Puerto Rican women go to clinics in the United States, they are treated like "crazy people," and their physical complaints are dismissed as only due to "nerves."[4]

Fatigue, Weakness, and Chest Pains

Approximately 25 percent of the women who come to Spiritist sessions, whose complaint profiles parallel those of mental health clients diagnosed with anxiety disorders, present with "fatigue" (including various forms of bodily weakness) and "chest or heart pains." According to the psychiatric manual (APA, 1987), these symptoms may be part of a "panic disorder" within a syndrome of extreme motor tension and autonomic hyperactivity.[5] In Linda's case (recorded at a *centro* session), complaints of weakness in various parts of her body and a sensation of tightness in her chest were included in what Spiritist mediums "saw" (*videncia*) of her experience of distress. From their descriptions of her inner feelings of distress, it appeared to us that Linda's "nervousness" referred to a kind of restless agitation, still another way in which *nervios* is expressed.

Linda

A woman of forty-seven years, whose much-older husband had just passed away, Linda's complaints (which the medium "captured" within her own body) were weakness in her arms, chest, and heart; hot and cold flushes; tightness in her chest; pain and palpitations in the nape of her neck; numbness in her entire body; deep suffering; and nervousness. Her problems were openly discussed by the mediums working at the table as due to the fact that Linda's husband had died suddenly of a "brain attack" (*ataque cerebral* or thrombosis) and "did not say goodbye." The medium implied that the surprise of his death had unhinged Linda.

The mediums produced two *videncias* and a possession that focused on Linda. One *videncia* described a "spirit mounted on a horse, dressed in a white robe and hat—galloping, galloping. He comes and opens his hands as if he is going to give you something, which is that you will become involved in the spiritual field so that this spirit can withdraw." A second *videncia* revealed that Linda had "married because she couldn't hold back even a little longer and wait for an opportunity to study. She could not stand the trials of living at home." The *causa* spirit possessing a medium said, "I am at the side of my companion. I appear to be material, but I am not. They tell me that I am a spirit. But I want to tell you that I am at your side. I want to talk to you in an intimate way, although it is through an outside brain. I have to separate from you. My spirit is going to cleanse itself more each day in order to one day come and help you. But until then nothing will be able to help you, because you have me stuck on to you."

We discussed later how the images and the spirits all pointed to the shock and helplessness that Linda was described as feeling because of the suddenness of her husband's death. They also pointed out that Linda was a person who feels unsupported, having been overly dependent upon her husband to whom she is still strongly attached. The main direction of the spirits' interventions was the instruction that Linda should become a Spiritist medium; her husband's spirit would "develop" and become her principal *guía*.

If we were to label Linda's state of extreme distress as an anxiety disorder, it would appear that Linda has had two or three panic attacks and is also anxious much of the time. The attacks seemed to have been caused by her husband's death, but her "nervousness" is recognized by the spirits (through the mediums) as antedating that event. This is implied in the spirit evidence that she married an older man because she felt so insecure.

It seemed to us that Linda was experiencing an inner conflict of grief and anger over loss of the man she relied upon to support her in her generally "nervous" state. The spirit of her husband spoke through the medium, pointing out how "attached" he is to her. He implied that her complaints mirror those he himself suffered at the time of his death. The commonness of experiencing the symptoms of a loved one who has died from a myocardial infarction is discussed by Nemiah (1985), who describes how many bereaved people manifest chest pain, palpitations, tightness of the chest, difficulty with respiration, and subsequent numbness (due to hyperventilation). The mediums "see" that Linda must come to terms with her husband's spirit in order to be freed of the negative effects of his continued presence. They recommend that she tame his spirit through prayer—one route to involvement in spirit work. This case illustrates that "nervousness" as "symptomatic contagion" is still another dimension of a culturally patterned syndrome composed of both somatic distress and anxiety. Loss of a significant other in a relationship chracterized by great dependency is a potent stressor that may precipitate panic attacks. We thought that Linda's distress may not become chronic and at that time appeared to be effectively helped by Spiritist treatment.

Treatment of Anxiety Disorders and Nerves

The hierarchy of resort in seeking help in cases of *ataque de nervios* is illustrated in the following case presented by a Spiritist:

Juanita

Forty years old and the mother of three teenaged children, Juanita suffered pains in her head, chest, waist, and the heels of her feet for three years. She was also "sick from nerves" and had insomnia. She then had an "*ataque de nervios*" and of "diabetes" and went to the local hospital emergency room. Her symptoms were not relieved, and she was forced to stop working. She then sought help from a private physician, Dr. Reyes, in the metropolitan area and at the same time was being seen at the mental health center in her community. Even with these treatments, which consisted of control of her diabetic condition, tranquilizers (*pastillas de los nervios*), and supportive therapy, she could not find

> relief. It seemed that the doctors could only refer to problems with her husband (he had "abandoned" his family by walking out and setting up house with a younger woman) and her children as causing her illness. Even more distressing to her was that her children told her she was "crazy."
>
> In this sorry state, Juanita responded to a friend's recommendation to see a Spiritist in their community, Doña Georgie. Juanita accompanied this woman to *centro*, though with great trepidation because this was her first experience. She was the first to be called to the table, and three *causa* spirits were lifted off of her. She returned the following week, and the "work" continued; baths were prescribed. She told assembled mediums and other participants that she felt better, having slept well for the first time in years. She also received *despojos* (cleansing of negative spirit influences by rotating movements of the arms around the upper body).

Doña Georgie (the presenter) said she "saw" that another woman had come between Juanita and her husband, and this woman had sent "bad thoughts" that penetrated Juanita's weakened defenses. These were countered at the session by the *despojos* and prayers. Soon afterward, Juanita's husband miraculously returned home, and her daughter, who had bitterly fought with her father, prompted by her mother, decided to make peace with him. Juanita then finally got relief from her "nerves" and "physical pains."

We noted that the criterion of "help" for Juanita was that she *felt* relieved, an experientially based assessment. Interestingly, control over her diabetes was not even mentioned as an issue.

Successful Spiritist treatment of mild phobic behavior can be appreciated in the following brief case description presented by another Spiritist healer.

Laura

> Twenty-eight years old, married seven years and the mother of four daughters, Laura and her physician husband had recently purchased a house in which a doctor had died. During these two months Laura frequently saw this man's ghost. She spent her days in a tense and frightened state, especially upset as night drew near. To make matters worse, Laura's husband began coming home late, saying that he had to take a female colleague home.

The medium whom Laura had consulted told us that Laura had talked to her about her dissatisfactions in life. It seems that Laura's husband wanted a son, and Laura already felt tied down with too many children. She really wanted to pursue her studies, which were put aside when she married and became pregnant. She felt trapped by inner conflict over her own lack of self-determination. Should she follow her husband's needs or her own? The medium prescribed prayers and readings and told Laura that she was "developing faculties" to see into the spirit world. She also said that "someone was jealous" of Laura's marriage and so had caused the doctor's spirit to appear in her home. But this *prueba* (test) was part of her "development." The medium then held several sessions in Laura's house as a kind of exorcism in which molesting spirits were instructed to leave Laura alone. Being told that someone envied her situation and that she had "special powers" appeared to satisfy Laura's need for greater self-expression, and her anxiety abated (at least for the moment).

We feel we must add the observation that moderately severe cases of panic disorder, phobias, or generalized anxiety disorder (such as those of Irene and Fela) are also successfully treated by sensitive psychologists and psychologically aware doctors. In Puerto Rico it seems that people with severe anxiety disorders are eventually seen by mental health professionals, because the sufferer is unable to function normally. The treatments for anxiety disorders used by mental health professionals in the 108 cases of women were, in order of frequency, as follows: individual psychotherapy (in 61 percent of the cases), supportive therapy (22 percent), medication (unspecified type, 15 percent), group therapy (14 percent), and Mellaril (thioridazine, 13 percent). Explanations of the causes and courses of these disorders are clearly different across the three healing systems, as already illustrated.

Panic Disorder, Agoraphobia, and "Development" in Spiritism

The first case described in this chapter was that of Evangelina, who had been a "nervous person" (in her words) most of her life. Here I will give some details of her early years and her much later initiation as a Spiritist healer, which (according to her own evaluation) effected a kind of "cure" for her distress. As the reader will note, in this case the folk concept of "nervousness" (or its equivalents) does seem to describe her experience of an "anxiety disorder," one initiated by a severe panic attack. The term "*ataque de nervios*" was used by Evangelina to describe a severe episode. Although this suggests a one-to-one equivalence of these terms (and categories), this is the exception rather than the rule. I repeat my hypothesis that "nervousness" is not directly equivalent to "anxiety" (defined as worry, tension) but does encode an experience of severe strain and vulnerability experienced as being within one's body.

Evangelina

Evangelina was the ninth of ten siblings born into a poor rural family. Their poverty seemed to have been so acute that she remembers seldom having a penny to buy a school lunch. She also recalls two terrible feelings toward her parents: they "rejected" her and they taught her fear and disgust toward sex. She has stayed single but has a "profound resentment towards them because of it." Moreover, she attributes her timidity and fear of strangers in part to the isolated life she felt her family led in the country during her childhood. She was forced to get a job at an early age, having only completed fifth grade; however, that was two grades more than her siblings had completed.

Evangelina took catechism classes and was a candidate for the "Daughters of Mary" society. (We might note that her early childhood did not appear to be as "isolated" as she felt it was.) When she was ten years old, for no apparent reason she began to have fainting spells. At fifteen she gave catechism classes to neighboring children, yet she would faint each time she went to church. Once when she felt very dizzy, she had a vision of the priest as the devil, complete "with horns and tail." In addition, she suffered from bronchial asthma during the years when she was nine to fourteen. The last time she had a fainting spell (when eighteen years old), she was praying for someone who had died. She "felt an odd sensation in her feet" and lost her sight. "Something" had bound up her chest. She then fainted. (This is a description of a "panic attack" according to the current psychiatric diagnostic criteria of at least four symptoms out of twelve [DSMIIIR, APA, 1987]. These symptoms are: dyspnea; palpitations; chest pain or discomfort; choking or smothering sensations; dizziness, vertigo, or unsteady feelings; feelings of unreality; tingling in hands or feet; hot and cold flashes; sweating; faintness; trembling or shaking; fear of dying, going crazy, or doing something uncontrolled during an attack.)

Evangelina said that at the time she had no knowledge that spirits attach themselves to people; later she interpreted the attack as caused by the dead person's spirit having become attached to her. On another occasion (after she learned about Spiritism), she went again to pray for a deceased individual. This time she heard the dead person say, "Look down." When she did, she saw a head on a plate. Later the spirit said, "This person will be next," and in three days the man whose head she saw died. Later, when Evangelina started work at a factory, she suffered frequent "attacks." One day she felt suicidal but prayed to God. She wanted to know if the devil was molesting her or if she was undergoing a test (*prueba*) from God. That very night she became possessed and heard only a *guía* speak. She described the Spirit as an old woman, dressed in a skirt and jacket from "ancient times." Her name was Amalia, and she earned her living as a laundress.

After this experience, Evangelina began to attend Spiritist sessions in many places. She subsequently suffered other episodes of illness, one of which she called an "obsession" (an overwhelming by a spirit and "craziness," with delusions and trembling). (This appears to have been another panic attack.) It was then that her family "attacked her verbally" and "threw her out." She moved in with the woman friend who continues to care for her, and after intensive work at a Spiritist session the obsession left. One day Evangelina received a message from a *guía* named Miguel Angel, who told her that she should form her own Spiritist study group. From that time forward (she was about thirty years old), she no longer suffered attacks but also said she worries that they might return.

We must note that although this appeared to have been the end of the attacks, Evangelina gradually developed other problems—she became extremely anxious about leaving home and even had difficulty accompanying her friend in the car. Dreams imaged the "inquisition pursuing her" while she was walking down a strange street. In another dream her friend told her to wait in the car and left. Shortly afterward men with guns entered the car, and one pointed a pistol at her head. They raped her, and her friend abandoned her. In a third dream her friend left her in the car on the bank of a dry river. The friend disappeared, and more and more people kept appearing. Evangelina felt "lost, confused, and afraid."

In our assessment, all of the previously-mentioned experiences seem typical of agoraphobia as described in psychiatric manuals such as the DSMIIIR. Moreover, the friend with whom Evangelina lives appears to accept this state of affairs and even reinforces her fears by vocally worrying about her on the rare occasions when Evangelina leaves the house with someone else. Their relationship is "rationalized" by Spiritist belief; Spiritists say that the friend persecuted and abandoned Evangelina in a former existence, and now her "test" is that she must protect and care for Evangelina in this one. Evangelina has never been seen by a mental health professional but had been treated in early adulthood by Spiritist mediums for the more severe panic attacks. She now seems to have adapted to her fears, coping with them through her friend, who is patient to an extreme and accompanies her everywhere. They lead a very home-centered life because they both stopped working more than ten years ago. They are supported by social security payments and fees for child care. Approximately ten years ago Evangelina established her own *centro* and does leave home regularly to preside over these sessions as well as to very occasionally attend others. According to her testimony, her emotional problems are rooted in early family experiences and fueled by pathological fears about sex and death. (She did not reveal whether she suffered sexual abuse during childhood, but the hidden suggestions made us wonder.) We speculated that she may have developed (or imitated) a "worrying" cognitive style during childhood because of the privations she and her parents experienced, her asthmatic condition (which could be both cause and effect), and her parents' very strict moral injunctions against sexual thoughts and behavior, such as masturbation, referring to or touching a boy's or girl's genitals, or talking about sexual intercourse.[6]

The role of Spiritist treatment, first in relieving the panic attacks and later in alleviating Evangelina's state of extreme fearfulness through her "development" as a medium, is interesting to examine. As described earlier, Spiritism is almost unique among treatments for emotional distress in focusing directly upon death. It deals with the dead by providing ways in which the expected harmful effects of their spirits' becoming attached to living beings can be either eliminated, controlled, or redirected into positive channels, such as when molesting spirits are converted into *guías*. These practices apparently helped Evangelina recover from her out-of-control episodes (*ataques*) as her fears of death slowly subsided. However, other fears remain, as expressed in her current phobic behavior. One dimension of her worries might be described as extreme apprehension about moral transgressions related to sexuality (and the death penalty for them). Her fears seem to have lessened through her activities as a healer, because she does "good work," that is, according to the will of God. She also seems to have found a situation in which, according to what she implied, she can avoid sexual activity and still have a caring and protective partner. Although the relationship is clearly personally satisfying, the women fall under the stigma of suspicions that they are lesbians. Although Evangelina never directly denied this aspect of herself and her relationship with her live-in friend, neither did she "come out of the closet."

Conclusions and Further Observations

This chapter has described women's experiences of what have been diagnosed as "anxiety disorders" and similar kinds of disorders among clients of Spiritist mediums. It has also explored "*nervios*" and "nervousness" as culturally patterned symptoms (popular complaints or conditions) presented by many women sufferers of anxiety disorders and also by others who present to medical clinics with physical illnesses. These popular terms are also sometimes used to refer to illness in people who have not yet presented for treatment to mental health clinics or Spiritist *centros* or who do not accept the diagnoses of therapists, medical doctors, or healers. I have attempted to show that although there is much overlap in meaning, "nervousness" is not conceptually equivalent to "anxiety" as defined in psychiatry and psychology. It denotes instead a special type of stress concept, which I will describe presently.

Puerto Rican mental health professionals are trained to use the psychiatric diagnostic manuals developed in the United States in much the same ways as their North American counterparts. However, their patients' most frequent complaints are somewhat different from the symptoms listed as diagnostic criteria of various anxiety disorders. For example, therapists' patients frequently present with "hostility," "crying jags," and "hallucinations," in addition to "nervousness" and "intranquility." Because the complaint of "crying jags" is also frequent among depressed women, we have observed that there is an overlap between affective disorder and anxiety disorder labeling in therapists' diagnostic practices. In Chapter 7 I characterized depressive states as falling much more on the agitated than on the depressed side of the depression syndrome; it is often difficult to distinguish between them. Moreover, as in the experience of depression, some women suffering anxiety disorders also complain of hallucinations and delusions. Whether these complaints are associated with the depressed dimension of their disorder or with the common "intrusive thoughts" of most people with phobias is difficult to tease out from these case studies. Because "visions" and sensations of spirits are fairly common expressions of distress among Puerto Ricans, we might expect that they could accompany severe emotional disorder of any type.

Yet another complaint, "hostility," appears more frequently in reports of people diagnosed as suffering from an anxiety disorder (approximately one-fourth) than in those of people diagnosed as dysthymic (approximately one-sixth). Here again we note that Puerto Ricans commonly release angry and aggressive feelings at highly stressful times. This complaint seems to reflect the way women tightly suppress their negative feelings until such time as their emotions are so chaotic that they lose control over them. Even when they report angry or aggressive feelings, a certain thinly veiled satisfaction appears that connotes a sense of "getting away with it." Yet anger and aggression in women most often stay at the verbal level and are rarely acted upon, except during psychotic episodes. However, in a few cases labeled *ataque de nervios* (or *obsesión*) by the Spiritists, women did become physically violent against themselves or others.

Complaints of "hostility," "crying jags," and "hallucinations" are not common in psychiatric literature on anxiety disorders. This supports the notion that culture makes a contribution both to the nature of anxiety disorders among women in Puerto Rico and to the construction of their illness behavior. Good and Kleinman (1985:321) comment that "anxiety disorders are not merely results of culturally influenced interpretations of an underlying disease; anxiety disorders are also disorders of the interpretive process." One's task doubles when analyzing cultural components of anxiety disorders, as these authors so clearly point out, because both disordered cognition and affect are integrally related to their genesis and course. Culture inevitably structures pathologies of interpreting and feeling, as well as supplying idioms of distress, illness concepts, categories, and models for responding to the inner experiences of emotional chaos and disordered perception.

An analysis of spirit intervention in the fifty cases that parallel anxiety disorders seen by Spiritist healers revealed particular themes. Spirits warned sufferers about the following prospective difficulties: illness or operations, craziness, harm (undefined), family conflict, and marital breakup. Frequent images brought to the sessions by spirits (in possessed mediums) were smoke, black or rotten water, blackbirds, wheelchairs, crutches, and spider webs. It is curious that the harm Spiritist clients were being warned about seemed to echo their worst fears about suffering bodily harm, being abandoned, or becoming crazy. The images reflected the same concerns as did the spirit warnings but also pointed to feelings of entrapment (the spider web) and of puzzlement and confusion (smoke, black water, blackbirds). Moreover, spirit evidence reported by mediums to clients (*videncias*) focused on three themes:

the sufferer feeling trapped, being muffled by a spirit (blinding or confusing her), or being in development (in which all of these feelings are common).

In our opinion, these metaphors express a quality of experience of inner disorder typical of what psychiatry labels "anxiety disorders." But they also describe the ways fears are constructed, as well as their content. Although there are other variations, these central fears highlight feelings about the body and the social self.

According to our "reading" of the case narratives, the way fear is expressed in both therapist and Spiritist cases (but especially in the latter) is better described by the concept of "worry" than by the concept of "anxiety." "Worry" is defined by Borkovec as a "chain of negatively affect-laden, relatively uncontrollable thoughts and images," brought on by objects or events associated with fear (1985:466). The chronic worrier tries to mentally solve the problem; the outcome is not only uncertain but contains primarily negative (harmful) possibilities. Moreover, highly distressed worriers seem unable to cope with the feared issue in an effective, action-oriented way. Spiritism seems to be an effective therapy for "worriers," because it both validates fears about negative outcomes (that is, labels and details the malaise) *and* converts the fears (commonly, sensations of bodily distress perceived as life-threatening) into means (for example, existential tests, *guías*) for achieving positive results. Thus Linda is told that the spirit of her dead husband, instead of continuing to inflict both physical and emotional pain, can become a supportive, protector-guide. Similarly, the "bad thoughts" sent by the woman who wanted Juanita's husband and caused her pain and "nerve sickness" could be taken off by a medium whose power countered that of the spirit sent to harm Juanita. (And, we must note, once she was less "crazy," Juanita's husband seemed to feel more comfortable at home.)

Finally, I again take up the question of what *nervios* "means" for Puerto Rican women. In the context of the cases previously described, "nervousness" primarily reflects bodily malaise. "Body," as I am using the term here, includes the head, brain, and mind. This kind of inner distress almost completely disorganizes both thought and behavior, resulting in feelings of confusion, lack of control, and ultimately the fear and actualization of bodily harm. The idiom "nervousness" can be thought of as equivalent to the concept of "stress" as popularly used in the United States, except that it represents an internal experience similar to what is commonly meant by the expression, "I feel stressed." "Nervousness" for Puerto Rican women appears to be a first cousin to the popular Mexican idiom of distress, "*asustado*" (frightened), which is also a part of the discourse on distress of Puerto Ricans, although used much less frequently. Rubel and colleagues (1984) showed *asustados* to have more disease signs and symptoms than matched controls, as well as higher rates of morbidity; their illnesses were also more life-threatening. Like "fright" in Mexico, "nervousness" in Puerto Rico connotes vulnerability to illness of all kinds—physical, emotional, psychiatric, or spiritual.

Notes

1. Pandolfi (1990:263–265) presents an interesting approach to understanding context and causality of vulnerability to illness in women. She suggests "two forms of expression that link collective history to that of each individual woman. One expression repeats a heritage of symptoms in the maternal line." The other is a "translation of events into an individual, fragmented somatic ritual." She specifies the second form as "history petrified in [particular] bodily features." Certainly these two forms of expression can be appreciated in the narratives about the experiences of suffering presented in this book. However, two caveats are necessary. First, the Spiritists as healers are those most likely to deal with collective history in general and heritage in particular. Their clients (much more often than patients of therapists) may use that form of expression but not at all in a systematic way, except, perhaps, in the area of conflict with traditional roles and role expectations. Second, as Pandolfi infers but does not specifically state, once the experience is focused within the body, outer events increasingly seem to shrink in importance, distanced by what she calls the "third level," the "deep personal corporeal experience." In the healing systems with which I am concerned in this book, the "deep corporeal experience" is either dealt with through invasive therapies, such as medications, or, in the case of the Spiritists, by reconstructions of past life events *felt* as deep within one's identity or sense of self as if these past events were transferred out of the body.

2. Differences between expectations for public and for private spheres of behavior and between gender roles complicate this observation. Aggressive behavior does seem to "leap out" spontaneously in many public arenas, mostly in men but occasionally in women. It erupts in the private arena as well (that is, in the family environment) where loss of control and peace are disapproved of to a much greater extent. However, if it remains hidden from the world, abusive behavior is much less likely to be subjected to sanctions and control. Many women collude in hiding abuse in Puerto Rico, as elsewhere. Although it is almost impossible to compare across cultures, I would speculate that the public and private spheres are kept more separate in Puerto Rico than elsewhere and that therefore abuse is more often hidden.

3. Toward a further understanding of these comparisons between men and women who present as "nervous" or "intranquil," we note that Canino and colleagues (1988) report fairly high rates of comorbidity between anxiety disorders and other psychiatric illnesses in Puerto Rico. Thus many "nervous" men may have additional psychiatric problems.

4. This may reflect non-Puerto Rican doctors' inability to "decode" certain complaints and attend to psychosocial problems underlying somatic expressions of distress.

5. Canino and colleagues (1987b) list chest pain as the second of the five most common panic symptoms, which also include palpitations, fear of dying or going crazy, choking, and sweating. Using responses to the Diagnostic Interview Schedule study (described in Chapter 6; Canino et al., 1987a), Guarnaccia and colleagues (1989b)

include "periods of weakness" and "chest pain" in a hypothesized scale of symptoms that characterizes "*ataques de nervios*" as equivalent to panic disorder.

6. Researchers hypothesize that an "anxiety-relevant cognitive style" composed of habitual catastrophizing, a focus on cues of danger while always screening out cues of safety, and obsessive holding on to intrusive, upsetting thoughts is etiological to agoraphobia and other phobias (Beck, 1976). Superimposed upon these cognitive distortions, Evangelina may then have developed exaggerated appraisals of the degree of danger associated with her panic attacks (Ganellan et al., 1986), leading to full expression of her present phobias.

The complete etiology of her distress is not known to us, but we were aware that Evangelina was not revealing the extent of her early trauma. We suspected that she had been abused sexually by some relative, because this is frequently encountered in this type of clinical picture, as other clinical case material in our experience shows.

10

Somatic Styles, Bodily Ills, and Somatoform Disorders

Not only does a person's representation of his own body influence his clinical symptoms, but the science which is then fashioned to "interpret" these symptoms itself constitutes a psychological representation of the human body which, once it is published, diffuses within a culture and becomes the basis of still further changes in the social representation of the human body.

—Robert M. Farr, *Indigenous Psychologies*

The overarching theme of this chapter is the body's role in the experience of emotional distress, which medicine classifies as organic, psychological, or psychosomatic in nature, and Spiritism classifies as either "material" or "spiritual." I am especially concerned with the ways women present and represent their bodies to the three types of healers who are the focus of this book. I am also intrigued with the converse—how women's bodies are represented and dealt with by the healers. The healers, depending upon their concepts, training, and personal experience, provide differing interpretations of the meanings of somatic complaints. Experience of one's body is especially important to Puerto Rican women as a gauge with which to assess the state of the "vessel" that provides them entry into those vital relationships through which they become wives and mothers. The bodies of women carry and convey highly charged meanings, leading to both general and physical expressions of distress through somatic idioms. Both positive and negative aspects of sexual experience and both gratification and denial of maternal nurturing tasks are reasons for expressing distress in bodily terms. Negative affects associated with facets of women's roles are in turn related to illness experience. They are sometimes directly expressed by presenting complaints such as vaginal pain but more often they are expressed by ambiguous symptoms that relate to unwanted sterility or lack of gratification in marital or maternal roles. Just as Kirmayer (1987) reports for his sample, women in Puerto Rico seem to feel more emotionally vulnerable than men; they also appear to be more vigilant in relation to bodily feelings.

"Somatization," defined in medicine and psychiatry as complaints about the body in the absence of demonstrable organic pathology (and including distressing perceptions of physical change in the body), is at the center of a current debate about how culture represents, patterns, and even displaces the expression of affect, especially dysphoric affect (Kleinman and Kleinman, 1985). Some observers note that verbal/categorical descriptions of distress tend to distance the sufferer from his or her experience of the emotions and feelings that are at the heart of the illness. The reader will soon see how difficult it is to sort out what is "somatization," given the cultural patterning of the communication of distress found among Puerto Rican women. Interior states are not displaced or expressed by somatic ones. As Kirmayer (1987) points out, "Worldwide, sociosomatics, which directly link social and somatic events, is a more common form of affective expression than the labelling of emotions as intrapsychic states" (1987:133).

In a comprehensive discussion, Kirmayer (1984b) describes seven "models" of somatization, not all of which are associated with illness: (1) result of attention focused on the body, (2) use of the body for communication, (3) an idiom of distress or way to give meaning to suffering, (4) a route to the sick role, (5) a concomitant of an affective (mood) disorder (or any psychiatric illness, but particularly depression, anxiety states, and addiction), (6) a result of how the health care system defines patienthood, and (7) a result of an incapacity for, or suppression of, emotional distress. Models (6) and (7) are especially associated with belief in the separation of mind and body as distinct sources and sites of disease, which is espoused by medical doctors and many mental health professionals. In contrast, as mentioned earlier, the important distinction for Spiritists is between body (*materia*) and spirit. In the discussion to follow, aspects of all of these models are used in attempting to understand women's perspectives toward their bodies and how women as patients and clients experience and represent distress through both somatic idioms and body-emotion transactions related to illness.

As described in preceding chapters, the complaint profiles that typify the experience of emotional distress (composed of eight general "diagnostic" categories) all include frequent somatic complaints (see Appendix, Table A.1). Of 753 naturally occurring complaints (before categorization) presented by all patients and clients, 365 directly referred to the body. The reader will note that particular complaints and their relative frequencies differ significantly across all categories, both among women as patients and between women and men (see Appendix, Tables A.1 and A.2). This provides evidence that naturally occurring complaints are basic units of a culturally patterned language of distress, each possessing multiple meanings (Nichter, 1981). Somatic complaints that refer to particular organ systems or general body states and feelings are important elements of this language among Puerto Ricans. For example, as was discussed in Chapter 7, in relation to depression and dysphoria, references to head pains seem to *mean* distress severe enough to be labeled illness. Certain conditions of the body—such as fatigue and weakness—in our interpretation of the narratives that include these complaints, commonly refer to feelings of hopelessness and apathy as well as to the inability to carry out social role requirements. (The weakness/tiredness syndrome will be described later.)

Sexual Socialization and Somatic References to Distress

In Chapter 6 I commented on the epidemiologic finding that psychosexual dysfunction is highly prevalent in Puerto Rico. Questions on the Diagnostic Interview Schedule, if unmodified by the clarification that in addition to "lack of interest," "lack of sexual desire" may or may not cause distress to oneself or to a partner, show that more than twice the number of women than men suffer from "psychosexual dysfunction" as defined by DSMIIIR criteria. For us, these data resonated with multiple (mostly indirect) references by healers, patients, and clients to their view that many women experience a kind of "turn-off" of their sexuality. We often discussed our perception that there are many ambivalences and paradoxes in sexual socialization that seem to affect sexual behavior among adults. These can be thought of as beginning with the very different attitudes parents have toward the male and female bodies of their children.

Such a difference in attitude is illustrated by the pride mothers take in their small sons' bodies and genitals. Some decades ago (and even now in some rural towns and *barrios*) small boys customarily went about unclothed, with their genitals exposed (Landy, 1959), although this custom is unusual in today's urban scene. A common exclamation when pointing to the genitals of a small boy is, "*¡Qué macho tú eres!*" (What a man you are.) In contrast, mothers are very concerned about covering up their small daughters' bodies, especially their genitals. Young girls are taught to protect their virginity from the ever-present *malicias* (evil ideas) of men and are absolutely required to learn virginlike behavior, such as sitting with their legs close together and covered, not roaming the streets by themselves during daylight hours, and staying at home at night unless escorted by an adult. Ideally, women—especially young women—are not supposed to be coquettish; yet their demeanor during their adolescent years loudly announces their desire to make up for the attempted suppression of sexuality during childhood. Masturbation and sex play among small children are equally denied to both sexes but occur much more often and are not uncommonly overlooked in boys. An uncomfortable paradox is repeatedly introduced and results from the attitude that it is highly desirable for women to marry at an early age—a goal that most young women have internalized. Thus adolescent girls receive an impossible message: marry young, but never pay attention to or flirt with young men!

We observed incest to be a special concern of many parents. They in fact work hard to keep male and female siblings physically separated in order to avoid any hint of bodily intimacy between them. Mothers are vigilant about their daughters' exposure to cousins, stepfathers, uncles, and other males but are not always successful. Although father-daughter incest accounts for most of the accusations and convictions we uncovered in legal records, such matters were rarely, if ever, discussed in the past (Hill et al., 1959). In fact, the reality of incest has only very recently begun to be discussed among mental health professionals.

In general, men do not consider it respectful to discuss sexual matters with their wives, nor do wives discuss such matters with husbands. And mothers rarely communicate with their nubile daughters about sexual matters. In contrast, many men are concerned that their fourteen- or fifteen-year-old sons be sexually initiated into manhood and may even shepherd them to the experience. Male cousins or uncles may find a prostitute or "loose" woman for them. Such attitudes and practices act as mixed messages between men and women; in our opinion, they seem to obstruct women's view of their own sexual feelings.

The paradoxical attitudes that sexuality is a taboo topic among family members and that sexuality is significant (and phenomenologically present in the family environment) are illustrated in the curious former practice of those parents who told riddles to their children at bedtime. Almost all of these riddles had obvious double meanings, the unacknowledged one referring to genitals or aspects of sexual intercourse. Of 227 examples published by Mason (1960), one, collected in the early part of the century, is a good example: "A little larger than a palm, as fat as it can be; charges and discharges in the hand of a woman." The official answer is "spindle." In my understanding of this bedtime ritual, reference to the sex act or genitals was never acknowledged. Indeed, children were supposed to give a sexually neutral (polite) answer. Although this customary way to "teach" sexuality has likely been replaced by bedtime television in most homes, its indirectness seems to remain as a prominent feature of the sexual socialization of children. They inevitably find out about the "facts of life" from older siblings and even more commonly from cousins or friends and the mass media.

But women seem to remain more or less under this taboo for most of their lives. From my participation in women's conversations, I noted that comments about the body were not common and were most often discussed in relation to illness or distress. Reproductive ailments were only vaguely mentioned and then only among women. I also noted that apart from sexual or reproductive references when communicating about distress, women and men seem to represent their bodies in very "natural" ways. They do not commonly talk about their bodies among themselves, and they do so even more rarely in mixed company. However, when they do refer to bodily functions, such as elimination or eating patterns and their effects, women seem to regard such themes as natural and not subject to restraint in conversational modes. And even though death and birth are fully accepted as "natural," in the past husbands and wives rarely discussed sexual matters (Landy, 1959). In one study, only 50 percent said they spoke about sexual matters at all, including planning for children (Hill et al., 1959). Change has occurred in terms of media messages, and some recent fiction by women refers to sexual intercourse without describing the act itself (see, for example, Vega and Lugo Filippi, 1981).

In amazing contrast to the strict rules that govern sexual relationships, an ambience of sensuality pervades many social settings. It reigns in most institutions—schools, offices, and so on—where there is frequent flirting among men and women, largely initiated by men but certainly assisted by some women. This sexualized *ambiente* in Puerto Rico is counterbalanced by rules that try to enforce sexual distance between unmarried women and their pursuers. Married women are less prey to male *malicias*, but divorced women are considered fair game. Moreover, there is unsuccessful reliance on individual compliance as well as patent omission when rules regarding sexual behavior are not observed. And although infidelity in marriage is strongly disapproved of, anecdotally at least, it occurs fairly frequently. Yet many women express ambivalence about sexual relations, even within marriage. In our opinion, this is in part because of the virgin-whore dichotomy in which women and men believe, and in part because men generally control both the opportunity for sexual experience and how and where it will occur.

In our view, a distressing confusion reigns when women are expected to be chaste while chased and at the same time taught that men are constantly looking to them for ways to prove their manliness. Societies that advocate the ideal of virginity for women and focus on male identity as partly achieved through sexual activity usually provide "loose women" and prostitutes to deal with this contradiction. The "woman-of-the-streets" image provides a stigmatized example for the many young women who can be caught by the pressing sensuality of young and middle-aged men. The former are very possessive and quick to feel anger and jealousy; but the latter are often equally quick to take advantage of a fresh young virgin. Women fear becoming pregnant out of wedlock and losing their chance at a socially advantageous marriage. This in part explains the long *noviazgos* (engagements), sometimes lasting from girlhood at thirteen years of age to marriage at twenty-one years of age or later.

Although we did not want to stretch our interpretation too far beyond the realms illustrated by the narratives, we privately queried whether certain somatic complaints are displacements of sexual conflicts and tensions. From a psychoanalytic perspective, the transposition of the image of the penis into a "spindle" in a woman's hand (in the previously mentioned riddle) appears to refer to the neutralization and domestication of sexuality, (literally) "in women's hands." And, as mentioned in Chapter 2, it is the disparaged "spinster" who is ideally sexually untouched; thus only she is able to control the "charge" and "discharge."

The preceding discussion describes aspects of attitudinal and social contexts for the deep, often fearful feelings that some women express about their bodies, as can be appreciated in the case narratives recounted later in this chapter. We observed that a common concept about the body in relation to health and illness is that health is equated with a strong body and illness with bodily weakness. Complaints such as "weakness in the head (brain)" or in a part of the body such as the arm or in both the "body and mind" are frequent in the case narratives we recorded. We deduced from them that the underlying meaning of "weakness" is a psychological incapacity to perform expected tasks and adequately carry out basic social roles.

Comparative Views of Body and Healing: Doctors and Spiritists

Spiritists have their own concepts about the body, which they described to us on numerous occasions and referred to frequently. They said they believed in a "physiological body," an envelope for an eternal spirit being who inevitably cycles through personal trials and incarnations until it is perfected and able to progress to the realm of the Holy Spirit, God. One's own spirit is identified prior to reincarnation in a material body, its personal identity forgotten upon the death of a prior material body. Spiritists also refer to the *periespiritu*, a "spiritual body" (also sometimes called the *psicosoma* or *cuerpo energético*). The *periespiritu* is not directly visible to anyone, including mediums, but it mirrors the physical body and is the actual target of Spiritist healing work. Healers must learn to capture or form an image of the *periespiritu*, because it cannot be seen directly. One medium compared it to the notion of "spiritual body" as described in the Bible in the book of Paul. Disencarnated spirits (either *guías* or *causas*) work on the *periespiritu* while a client sleeps. This structure links body and spirit and acts as a "shock absorber" for spirit influences affecting the body.

We observed how frequently mediums consigned clients' physical bodies to medical doctors and minimally directed their treatments to them. Apart from prescribing herbal teas and baths (most aimed at tranquilizing anxious clients), mediums worked mainly on the *periespiritu*, which they said is both a "mediator" and an *enlace*, a "link" between body and spirit. Various "exotic" healing techniques, such as psychic surgery and treating someone at a distance (all you need is an image of their body, not the *materia* itself), might be better understood if the presence of the *periespiritu* is taken into account. In addition, some healers said that they were able to "see" the biohistorical record of a client's incarnations. Juana, for example, described such a case:

> Beside this woman I see a personality. She [the client] can say "Well, look, that is my grandmother, that is my friend, my father" and can give all the characteristics. Why? Because that body preserves the characteristics of the spirit in its last incarnation. A medium is able to see other forms of the energetic body, like someone who looks at an album going backward in time and recognizes figures and past lives.

In contrast, Dr. Ortiz, a psychiatrist who participated in the Project, presented the case of a fifty-one-year-old woman, who he said complained excessively but did not have demonstrable organic pathology. Apparently paraphrasing his medical textbook (or so we thought), Dr. Ortiz reported:

> The body is an imperfect machine that readjusts, adjusts, and on top of that we maltreat it because of some hot tidbits that we throw into an empty stomach. Then we put in two aspirins, we give it a shot of rum; we do whatever, we diet five days, and this poor stomach is closing. What happens? We suffer its ajustments and its readjustments, and in a given moment they can cause pain and difficulties. It isn't a disease, it's a readjustment of the body. Not everyone needs to be a doctor in order to know it's a readjustment, and most people don't give the body time to end its readjustment and learn that the pain will end (without medical treatment).

Dr. Ortiz further acknowledged that these "illnesses" are relieved by doctors but also are relieved without their help. He commented that "doctors view treatment as only symptomatic, based on what physicians invent for these cases." Despite training in psychiatry Dr. Ortiz never mentioned a connection between the sufferer and psychological or social aspects of her illness. He seemed to insist that without positive results from laboratory tests, there was no pathology. The possibility of what is now called "somatization disorder" (formerly "hysteria" or "conversion reactions") did not seem to occur to him at that time. We noted that this interpretation of a patient's distress was opposite to that of Spiritist healers. Because Spiritists have a heightened sensitivity to the body-spirit relationship, as well as a fear that they will get into trouble if they are not sure about the etiology of an illness, their practice has been traditionally to refer to medical doctors. They frequently advise a client that "You need a checkup." The basic difference betweeen doctors and Spiritists, apart from very different notions about the etiology of somatic distress, is the refusal of many doctors to look at somatic symptoms as meaningful symbols of distress emerging out of interpersonal situations.

In contrast to the medical doctors, we noted that Spiritists used bodily symptoms for diagnostic and treatment purposes and rarely used them in the service of a verbal exegesis of the illness or problem. Spiritists seemed to view somatic complaints as parallel to (but not substitutes for) affective states or as symbols of them, as well as metaphors for difficulties in relationships between living people and between spirits and living people. Equating somatic complaints with affects (but also at times highlighting the lack of relatedness between them) is a key element of diagnosis and the healing process for Spiritists. Their general approach is to transfigure negative emotions, first by distancing them from the sufferer (by taking them into their own bodies) and then by transforming them into feelings and emotions with positive valences (Koss, 1986, and Chapter 4).

It is of considerable interest that none of the three types of healers—medical doctors, Spiritists, and mental health professionals—seems to favor the type of treatment that subordinates clients' and patients' feelings and emotions to verbal descriptions. Our observations suggest that psychiatrists and medical doctors operate mostly within a Puerto Rican pattern of expression of emotion, which is largely nonverbal, gestural, and phenomenological, rather than within a prescribed biomedical pattern, which is largely verbal, abstract, and categorical. For healers and other Puerto Ricans, experience is valued for itself rather than as an example of a psychological state upon which one might reflect or which one might even treat.

Diagnostic Categories and Case Narratives

Undiagnosable Cases ("Deferred Diagnosis")

In addition to the ideas and events provided by the ninety-one therapist (mental health workers and medical doctors) and twenty-five reclassified Spiritist cases in the large, computer-analyzed sample, this discussion uses two cases from the case review sessions and two from individually collected case studies in order to explore the nature of "deferred cases" and how these particular patients and clients are treated. The therapists, doctors, and Spiritist healers who saw these patients and clients did not diagnose them in any specific way. We felt that these cases were especially important to explore because they represented about one-third of all cases seen by Spiritist healers, most of the clients having self-referred after unsatisfactory experiences in medical clinics. We commented privately that these cases illustrated therapists' confusion about what kinds of distress were present—somatic or psychologic. With regard to the Spiritists, the traditional choice of location and cause of distress is a simple one—between body and spirit. They seemed to hedge their bets when confused about the nature of the illness by sending the client to a doctor *and* working with them spiritually at the same time. In other studies, we had observed that before participating in the Project, the Spiritists rarely, if at all, referred to mental health professionals. The few exceptions were in regard to severely disordered patients whom they were unable to render calm enough to treat.

We heard many variations on the theme of a patient suffering somatic complaints feeling rejected by medical doctors who, after many lab tests with negative results, said they could not help the patient. A few doctors would suggest that the patient consult a traditional healer, but most simply gave the patient the impression that she must seek help elsewhere. The doctor would sometimes be reported to have said something like, "Your condition is in God's hands." The following case, presented by a Spiritist healer, who reported her client's feelings and views, illustrates this pattern. In our experience, it is a typical example of a patient's perception of a physician who became frustrated when all of his research failed to find a physical cause for her discomfort. The Spiritist healer specifically commented on the fact that the doctor failed to include psychosocial factors in his consideration of the cause of the patient's distress.

Elvira

> Elvira, a woman of forty-five years, suffered from "high fever, vomiting, diarrhea, inability to eat, and recent weight loss." She went to her doctor, who sent her for multiple laboratory analyses: urine, blood, and stool, as well as chest and kidney X rays and other kidney studies and a PAP test. He prescribed some medicine. I think it was Valium. All the lab tests were negative, but Elvira's fever continued and she lost weight at a rapid pace until she weighed only seventy-five pounds. The doctor told her, "I can't go on with you; go to one of those *Espiritistas*, go to a *curandero*, or go to a witch." A cousin who was with Elvira when the doctor told her these things suggested she visit the *centro* of Doña Carla "for medicine."

Doña Carla said she recommended baths of medicinal plants and teas of the herb molinillo (*Hura crepitans*) to be taken in the morning before eating (molinillo is used for fever). However, the focus of the treatment was a spirit, which was inadvertently causing her distress. The mediums at the *centro* discovered that this was the spirit of a close friend of Elvira, who had recently died of cancer. The friend's spirit was looking for help from Elvira. While the friend was dying, Elvira could not attend to her because she was preoccupied with her paralyzed husband and two small daughters.

Doña Carla commented that Elvira's complaints did not stop until she had taken a series of teas and attended sessions at the *centro* on several nights.

However, Elvira reported to us that the doctor's medications may also have been involved in her cure. She assured her interviewers that he was a "great doctor"; "he just didn't find the key to my problem." Moreover, she said that what she had "wasn't the doctor's" (that is, it wasn't primarily a physical illness).

Curiously (to us), many of the mediums at this case review session wanted first to verify Elvira's age. Later, we were privately told by one that they wanted to know if she was menopausal; they alluded to her concern about her friend's death as related to fears about her own mortality. The mediums then made references to her difficult family situation, seeing it as germane to their notions about how "stress" entered into Elvira's illness. The somatic problems were seen by them as metaphors for feelings, emotions, and concerns; that is, they saw Elvira's pain and severe distress as signs of the serious illness of her close friend incorporated into her *periespiritu* (body-spirit link) rather than as being symptomatic of her own body's illness.

We discussed the notion that if we saw Elvira's malaise through a psychiatric lens, this case might look like a "somatization disorder" as defined in the Diagnostic and Statistical Manual (APA, 1987). However, Elvira reported that she was "cured" of her somatic complaints; she did not continue to manifest these or others following her Spiritist treatment and her visits to the doctor. We noted that there is a significant difference in how practitioners in these different healing systems conceive of the body: in biomedicine, signs and symptoms are references to the body, but little more; in Spiritism, signs of distress and complaints seen as "evidence" can be many things. Somatic complaints are interpreted (and experienced) as being both in the body *and* in feelings about the body but also as signs of inner and outer distress in both the interpersonal and spiritual life arenas. Thus the Spiritist belief that certain illnesses are contracted from ill spirits is also a metaphor for how emotions affect the expression of somatic symptoms. Elvira felt badly that she had neglected her friend when she was dying, and she felt guilty. She also seemed to anticipate anger from her friend. In this way somatic symptoms are more than bodily complaints or fears about personal illness—they are also idioms of distress over conflictual feelings and incorrect moral behavior.

We observed that the narrative of another Spiritist case illustrated the absolute lack of distinction between what medicine labels "psyche" and "soma." This was the case of a woman who suffered for years from asthma. Her illness was labeled by the Spiritists as "*fatiga emocional*" (emotional weariness or hard breathing caused by emotion). Although treated medically for a number of years, the patient was certain that her "cure" had come from her visits to *centros*, under whose aegis she gradually developed as a medium. What seemed clear to the Spiritists was that the ultimate cause of her illness was "emotional" rather than physical. We observed that for believers in Spiritism, feelings and emotions are both embodied and embedded in a personal/interpersonal realm. In order to deal with this two-dimensional realm of experience, Spiritists regularly try to transcend it, that is, go beyond ordinary social events to its beginnings and endings, in other words, to the spirit world.

Still another case presentation illustrated to us how Spritism displaces medical concepts about psyche-soma relationships in illness by casting them into a transpersonal dimension of experience. However, Spiritism also has a distinct conceptualization of how interpersonal distress is embodied.

Anita

> A woman of thirty-two years, Anita presented with distress over her inability to carry a pregnancy to term. She had had two ectopic pregnancies in the prior year but finally gave birth to a son, then eighteen months of age. At the heart of her pain was a fear that the man with whom she lived would seek custody of his child and then leave her. (We must point out that this is the same issue we discussed in the chapter on depression, that is, women's deep concern with their reproductive capacity as the sine qua non of their identities as wives and women.) Her live-in partner was married to another woman and deaf to Anita's pleas that he divorce and marry her. Anita said she felt that the failed pregnancies were her punishment for the moral irregularity of her relationship and this would bring further pain.

We discussed how in this case the "illness" seemed to be experienced as failure of the body and was seen to be the result of moral turpitude. This meant that only Spiritists or other religious healers could effectively deal with it. In our observation, this reflects a deep sense of the notion (common in Puerto Rico and other Hispanic countries) that one's body is ultimately under God's control. Only by appealing to Him can a remedy be found.

The following case presentation illustrates how Dr. Ramirez, a medical doctor, initially failed to attend to either the psychological or the psychosocial aspects of her patient's experience of distress.

Flavia

> Flavia was eighteen years of age. She was diagnosed as having cystitis and a severe urinary tract infection. According to Dr. Ramirez, this was "rare" in one so young. The girl was hospitalized for a week, treated with an antibiotic, a pain killer, and a tranquilizer and released. However, a week later Flavia reappeared with the same complaint. She then told the doctor that she had been a medium for two years while in New York. She said that she was covered with a "white mantle," that is [in her interpretation], she was vulnerable to "bad works" being carried out against her. But Dr. Ramirez went through her routine medical workup without paying any more attention to Flavia's symbolically pointing to a need for "protection" in light of her self-diagnosed vulnerability to illness and stress.

Dr. Ramirez was an avid participant in the Project and when presenting the case of Flavia, she realized that Flavia's descriptions of the source of her malaise had some significance and so reported them to the group. But she had been unable to relate this symbolic expression to her view of Flavia's problem as an episodic, recalcitrant infection. Because Dr. Ramirez did not take a complete social history and because we were unable to interview this woman, we never found out what events preceded Flavia's bout with cystitis. We speculated that they might be similar to those in the case of Elvira, that is, due to the intrusion of a dead friend's spirit. From Elvira's perspective, the death of her friend from cancer was a "near miss" as regards her own state.[1] We commented on the fact that Spiritist healers are probably the only sources of help available to people who feel vulnerable through death loss. Their healing methods always focus on the impact of death, and they serve to directly confront such traumatic events when they become embodied through a sense of vulnerability.

Physical Illness ("No Psychiatric Diagnosis")

Only a small number of the clients seen by Spiritist mediums were diagnosed as having complaints with strictly organic causes, and these clients were immediately referred to medical doctors. The case of Niña is a good example of the certainty mediums exhibit when making this type of diagnosis.

Niña

> At a *centro* session Niña, a women of sixty-five years, was told to stand. She was asked by the head medium if she had an appointment for an operation. When she replied no, the medium told her, "I have seen an admission to the hospital for a vaginal exploration. Even though you don't have an appointment, you feel a hot sensation in your vagina, your stomach is swollen, your legs are numb, there is also vaginal burning. Your eyes fill with tears, you feel sharp pains in your eyes, your nose is stopped up, and your throat is dry." Niña then answered that all this was true. The medium became possessed, and the spirit said, "If you are ill, if you are seriously distressed, what are you doing here? Go to the hospital!" Niña trembled, "They won't help me in the hospital." The spirit [in the medium] then said, "You are rotten down there. Why do they tell me that I am the ill person? That I am forming the illness in your body? Whoever says it [does so] in the name of God. Thank you for having brought me here."

Watching this session, we then heard the head medium say that she had seen a doll in a coffin. Describing the vision she said, "She [the doll] has a crown upon her head. You [Niña] are carrying the coffin to the entrance of the cemetery." Niña then replied, "I haven't seen myself arriving at the doors of the cemetery, but I have seen the coffin with the doll." The medium was twice more possessed by the spirit molesting Niña, who finally confessed that the symptoms were his (the spirit's) fault. We thought that the reference to the coffin was clearly a suggestion about the seriousness of Niña's illness. Niña was being warned that medical treatment was urgent, a life or death matter. The doll represented Niña, both as a symbol of her neglect of her health and as a replacement for herself should she heed the spirit's words and seek medical treatment. The image of "the crown" was perhaps a sign that the doll also represented Mary, Queen of Heaven, as the sacred mother who was watching over Niña and who would save her from dying if she received medical treatment. (Later we found out that Niña did go to the hospital and a benign ovarian cyst was removed without serious consequences.)

Medical attitudes and a patient's response toward illness defined by doctors as psychosomatic were illustrated by the case of Agripina, a divorced woman of fifty years, living apart from her only son, whom we intervewed.

Agripina

Agripina said that she sought help at the area hospital following a severe attack of asthma that she attributed to having been in contact with flowers at the viewing of a dead friend. She had suffered many such attacks for more than twenty-five years and had been treated by many doctors in public health centers. However, she had no knowledge of the type of medication previously prescribed. She was hospitalized for this attack, and the doctor attempted to inquire about possible emotional factors, but all Agripina would say was that she felt lonely (a not unusual condition of divorced, lower-income women living in public housing projects). The doctor noted in the chart that Agripina acknowledged that she felt "nervous" but would not talk about her feelings.

When questioned about her concerns about Agripina, the doctor responded that she observed the patient to be "very nervous, anxious, fearful, with premonitions that something was going to happen." "She seemed extremely suggestible, appeared hypochondriacal, and was possibly superstitious." We had to note that, unable to get verbal statements from Agripina about how she was feeling and in order to verify a psychosocial contribution to the illness, the doctor supplied her own explanation. It is instructive that this type of patient is labeled as "superstitious," that is, Agripina was unable or unwilling to accept the doctor's model of her illness, even though she readily accepted the treatment. It is clear that Agripina, like many other women, defined her illness as "somatic" and therefore was unwilling to disclose her feelings and problems to the doctor.

Somatic Complaints and Long-Term Mental and Physical Illness

There are many discussions in the literature on U.S. populations about the fact that people with schizophrenia and affective disorders manifest frequent somatic complaints (see, especially, Katon et al., 1982). The most frequent complaints in the profiles of Puerto Rican women diagnosed with psychiatric illnesses are headaches, head and memory problems, fatigue, and sleep disturbances. Those with dysthymia frequently complain as well of heart and chest problems (see Appendix, Table A.1). Spiritist cases reclassified under all of these disorders have somewhat fewer somatic complaints than do the therapist cases, but somatic complaints referring to multiple body sites are scattered throughout all of the profiles. Spiritist clients commonly list as many as twelve complaints each, and a few as many as twenty-seven body complaints, many mixed with feeling complaints, such as "nervousness," the desire to "walk," and "bad humor," a reference mainly to "irritability."

In the case of María, a woman of sixty-five years suffering from chronic schizophrenia, her therapist interpreted her frequent somatic complaints as a secondary diagnosis, "conversion disorder" (defined in the DSMIIIR [APA, 1987:57] as an "alteration or loss of physical functioning that suggests physical disorder, but that instead is apparently an expression of a psychological conflict or need"). When María's therapist presented her case, the Spiritists questioned her way of dealing with María's somatic complaints, saying that both María's age and previous psychiatric treatment were important factors that contributed to the possibility that María's complaints might have an organic cause overlooked by the mental health clinicians treating her.

María

The therapist recounted that

> María was mother to twelve children and presently was living with one of her sons. She had been diagnosed as schizophrenic at about twenty-nine years of age and had been last hospitalized at fifty-one years of age. Each time she received some news about her children, she would enter into a catatonic state but had not done so for at least six years. She slept poorly, awakened in bad humor, was restless, and given to obscene language. In general, she was not "very communicative." Moreover, she complained of numerous stomach, head, and body pains, yet all lab tests were negative. María had no interest in anything but her children and complained if they did not visit but also if too many came at one time. [We speculated that this reaction might be due to difficulties with overstimulation commonly seen in people with schizophrenia.]

The Spiritist healers reviewing this case "captured" that the causes of María's illness were both material and spiritual: the latter was the result of spirits who had caused difficulties since her birth. One medium asserted that some tranquilizing medication given to María "with a needle" caused cerebral problems. They also insisted that she had been hospitalized because she "suffered from the impact of great anger" that had not been understood. It was suggested that her family become part of the treatment because her relationships with them affected her illness and her preception of what had caused it. (We noted that educating the family about a schizophrenic relative is an important tool in preventing relapse; see, for example, Falloon et al., 1981.)

We observed that the Spiritist healers seemed to view María's somatic complaints as a language of distress pointing to a sociosomatic dimension of María's illness that had not been considered in her treatment by the mental health clinicians.[2] The Spiritists were actually rejecting María's therapist's diagnostic premises, especially after the therapist reported that her patient did not perceive herself to be mentally ill but was brought in by a daughter. The mediums instead took a tack that emphasized the problems the elderly have in relation to the ambivalence of their grown children. They alluded to María's feelings of powerlessness, which, they observed, lay behind her lack of ability to communicate her needs and feelings. They were also willing to accept María's version of her distress as somatic and locate at least one large part of the "cause" in problematic familial relationships.

We noted that because Spiritists are able to look at cases of mental illness from a multidimensional perspective, their interpretation of the somatic leads to a more meaning-centered treatment approach, one that considers complaints as metaphors, especially if expressed by people who otherwise are unable to communicate about certain types of distress. In our view, the Spiritists were not referring to the disturbances and abnormalities of the cognition of mentally ill people but to the fact that their situations can limit their openness of expression about conflicts with relatives and even about their inner, personal distress. Spiritists point to the possibility that in these cases the complaints themselves are both evocative and communicative. In the case of María, it seemed impossible for her to express her distress over her childrens' treatment of her, given her dependency upon them and her fear of arousing their ready anger and annoyance built up over years of experiencing her former bizarre behavior. Al-Issa (1982) points to several studies of women with schizophrenia that show that they frequently present with sexual symptoms representing their dissatisfactions with sexual relationships.

Hilda

A therapist presented the case of Hilda,

> who expressed her symptoms as, "I feel dead in life because my vaginal organs are affected and are disintegrating" and "I have a vaginal infection" [although this complaint was persistent, there was no physical (laboratory) proof]. Hilda also complained of being physically abused by her husband and being forced to

have sexual intercourse with him against her will. However, there was no evidence of bruises or lesions.

It seemed clear to us that somatic complaints in such cases are considered by therapists as delusional and due to the not unusual cognitive distortions found in schizophrenic people. It is as if they experience the body as outside of their control, as part of the tendency to feel depersonalized. However, we had to point out to the assembled participants that Hilda's report could well be a "rational" explanation, given the fact that men dominate women's sexual lives and can be abusers of their wives. Hilda's expressions of distress may be delusional but their sociocultural context is real enough.

In contrast to their attitudes and views on chronic mental illness, Spiritists take a somewhat different stance in the face of serious physical illness, a stance that clearly separates body and spirit. As one Spiritist healer remarked, "If the person suffers from ulcers or a cancer, you say to her, 'You don't have cancer or whatever; your body has suffered this or that, but your spirit is completely healthy. Don't take this experience into your spiritual register because your spirit is clean; it doesn't have these conditions.'" This accords with the idea, frequently expressed, that the body is merely a temporal container on a journey that will be repeated until the trials it must undergo are completed and the spirit can forever reside near the Holy Spirit. We observed that in the cases where women believe they have a disease caused by spirits who themselves had the disease while incarnated, the body is seen by them as vulnerable because their own spirit is weak and unenlightened. However, once an actual separation of body and spirit is imminent (through death), the spirit is once again seen as strong and healthy, as it will be in its next incarnation.

Somatoform Disorders

Under the psychiatric category of somatoform disorders (APA, 1987) there are six separately labeled mental disorders. However, here I will focus on cases illustrating the three most frequently presented at our review sessions or recounted in interviews: "somatization disorder," "hypochondriasis," and "conversion disorder." It is often difficult to diagnose somatization disorders because they so closely resemble depression (particularly in Puerto Rico). In general, diffuse somatic complaints are often interpreted as substitutes for dysphoric affect (Katon et al., 1982). We saw evidence of this confusion in the case of Leticia, who was treated at a Spiritist center.

Leticia

A thirty-five year old woman, Leticia presented twenty-seven complaints [that is, these were "seen" by the mediums and confirmed by Leticia], of which fifteen referred directly to bodily discomfort and pain. These were headaches, strong vibrations in her heart, back pain, eyes burning, ears itching, a sensation of "heaviness," fatigue, lack of appetite, stomach discomfort, dryness, stabbing pains in her back, the taste of blood in her mouth, "blocking." Her remaining complaints were nervousness, a desire to cry, feelings of desperation, heaviness, tiredness, sleepiness during the day, insomnia, the desire to go far way, a desire to take her own life, restlessness, uneasiness, and sadness. [We noted that the diffuseness and length of the somatic complaint list are exactly what might lead to a diagnosis of somatization disorder if this pattern of complaining was present before the age of thirty and part of a belief in being sickly. But the second list is more typical of a pattern of complaints found in depressive disorders. (See Table A.1, in the Appendix to compare the two profiles.)]

Three diagnoses of cause demonstrated the mediums' perspectives on Leticia's problems. They saw that she was "in development" which meant that her emotional disorder was a serious, chronic condition. In addition, she had two *causa* spirits: a Hindu who practiced magic and was "far back in search of light," and another who had committed suicide in a prior existence.

We shared the thought that these *videncias* pointed to the healers' considering Leticia's suicidal intent as most important but also suggesting that her problems were tricky to deal with. In other words, her somatic complaints looked to them as if she were fooling herself. Our interpretation is corroborated by the fact that they did not refer her to a medical doctor and never even asked her if she was under a doctor's treatment. Later they told her that she must pray, have more faith in the spirits, read the Bible, reject her tears, "dominate" the invading spirits, and continue to attend *centro* sessions in order to "develop." Looking at these remedies, it seemed apparent that the mediums recognized that Leticia's somatic complaints were not due to organic causes, that her main need was to combat her depressive tendencies, and that her bodily malaise pointed to a chronic condition rather than an acute emotional problem.

We also noted that the presence of so many somatic complaints at different body sites without demonstrated organic pathology certainly suggests "somatization disorder" (in the DSMIIIR, APA, 1987, thirteen is the number of symptoms that would qualify a case for this diagnosis) as well as a diagnosis of depression. However, the healers did not ask if Leticia was seeing a doctor or was taking medication, criteria that are also necessary in making the diagnosis of somatization disorder. They simply "knew" by relying on the experiences of their own bodies that these complaints were not "material"; that is, they did not "capture" the physicality of Leticia's somatic complaints.

Fatigue, Tiredness, Weariness, and Weakness

The complaint profiles of somatoform disorders among Spiritist and therapist clients suggest that "fatigue" (including weariness and tiredness of the whole body or any part of it) is a key symbol in a semantic network underlying discourse about somatic complaints. We observed that these kinds of complaints actually refer to a state of mind, that is, the conscious or unconscious ability to carry out expected duties associated with familial and social roles. Sixty-nine percent of Spiritist clients reclassified as having a somatoform disorder complained of fatigue, tiredness, or weariness, as did 15 percent of therapists' patients. The meanings of this expression of distress seem to be widely shared, even if it is not presented as frequently in clinical settings as in Spiritist healing sessions. Among Spiritist clients who fall within several categories, complaints of fatigue and weariness are frequent (see Appendix, Table A.1). Yet "fatigue" as a complaint is fairly frequent (6 percent) only in those therapist cases categorized as "no psychiatric diagnosis." We discussed the notion that the popular interpretation of "fatigue" and "weariness" shares some elements with the psychiatric interpretation; that is, that patients' excessive and nonorganically based somatic complaints result from dissociated, unconscious wishes for "secondary gains." This is a state of sickness in which the sufferer can legitimately avoid expected tasks or relationships without social disapproval or receive attention otherwise unavailable to her. We felt that it also points to inner conflicts over losses related to her identity as a woman.

Lola

The narrative of Lola's illnesses illustrates how the Spiritists interpret and treat the problem of "fatigue" or "tiredness." Lola's experience centered on her reaction to menopause. This is a case presented by a Spiritist to a case review session. The therapists, both medical doctors and mental health professionals, avidly added their comments to explanations of the dynamics and cause of Lola's problems.

> A woman of forty-eight years, Lola was married with four children and two others she was rearing (*hijos de crianza*). Shortly after an ovary was removed, she felt intermittent but strong heart pains. A doctor told her that there was nothing wrong and prescribed tranquilizers. Another did the same. At the hospital an electrocardiogram was negative and a cardiologist confirmed that she was healthy and free of heart disease. Her heart "felt better," but she began to feel tired, her face became swollen, and she had chills. She continued to visit doctors, who seemed at a loss to explain her symptoms. At this point Lola's brother took her to a *centro* where she was "treated" by being put at the table next to the mediums. She was given some instruction, especially in meditation, and also treated with "magnetic passes." After Lola had attended the sessions for approximately six weeks, the head medium visited her home and both became possessed by the spirit of Lola's mother. Just after this spirit's surprising appearance, the spirit of a Dutch priest named Benedict came through Lola and

was extremely hostile. After the experience of being possessed by the spirits causing her distress, Lola continued to attend the *centro*, and her distress gradually subsided. However, she also continued to see doctors for her heart pains. Another cardiologist found "nothing wrong"; still another said that a vein was reduced in size, causing an oxygen insufficiency.

At this point Lola became aware that she sensed her mother's spirit's presence as soon as she felt heart pains. Her mother had died of heart disease some nine years before, and Lola was "very attached" to her. As soon as she felt her mother's presence, Lola suffered "vibrations" that were like "bad feelings." She also felt malaise, described as "fatigue," when the priest's spirit came close to her. A third spirit also began to affect her. A nun who had been run over by a motorcycle was transmitting severe back pains when Lola "felt" her presence.

The medium presenting the case said that Lola's mother was affecting Lola in this way in order to assist another daughter through her. (We thought that this seemed to be a way of describing the sisters' rivalry for their mother's attention as well as Lola's pain in relation to her mother's death because she could no longer try to get her mother's love.) The mother had been described by Lola as very religious (*una fanática*). The priest's anger and the nun's affect were interpreted by the medium as reflecting her mother's and her family's disapproval of her becoming a medium.

At this point in the case review discussion, a psychologist wanted to make the point that a psychodynamic approach was better than this medium's explanation of Lola's problems. The therapist advanced the Freudian notion that religious images represent inner discomfort over sexual matters. Another therapist commented, "With menopause a woman no longer feels like a woman." A doctor then countered, "But I have read that menopausal women have more capacity to enjoy sex." The psychologist in turn replied, "But not in Puerto Rican culture." The Spiritists reviewing this case then became interested in confirming that Lola was menopausal; they seemed to agree that the underlying reason for Lola's distress was her loss of the capacity to bear children. (We observed privately that menopausal women in Puerto Rico closely associate fertility with femininity and feel that they are "over the hill" once they lose their periods. This could account for a mixed picture of depression and somatization, given the deep feeling that the body can no longer serve as a positive source of identity and esteem. Loss of the "mother" capacity for Lola constellated thoughts about losing her own mother. It seemed to re*vive* old and deep feelings of longing, rejection, and competition.)[3]

The mental health professionals reviewing Lola's case diagnosed her as suffering from hypochondriasis, whose criteria as a psychiatric illness include "preoccupation with the fear of having . . . a serious disease, based on the person's interpretation of physical signs or sensations as evidence of physical illness" (APA, 1987). The manual also cites "appropiate physical evaluation . . . that does not support the diagnosis of any physical disorder" and that "the fear of having a disease persists despite medical reassurance." We were aware that in cases where doctors label an episode of illness as "hypochondriacal," their criteria are usually diffuseness of the symptom picture and frequent medical visits at which the patient asks for help with an ever-changing symptom picture.

Somatization and Delusions

We observed that Spiritists and therapists seem to agree on the etiology and dynamics of manifestations of somatic disorders that lack a physical cause but manifest only as bodily malfunction. In psychiatry these conditions are usually labeled "conversion disorders" and described as "a loss or alteration in physical functioning suggesting a physical disorder," but the symptom is "related to a psychological conflict or need" and is tripped by a timely psychosocial stressor. Moreover, the sufferer is "not conscious of intentionally producing the symptom" (APA, 1987:259). A rather rare case of false pregnancy (this also occurs in other cultural settings) presented by a therapist illustrates how such disorders are seen by Spiritists and therapists. The therapist presenting the case did not mention whether her patient was suffering from dementia, but the patient had been in treatment at the mental health center for over two years. (We forgot to ask this question at the time.)

Myrna

> An eighty-year-old participant in Project Hope, Myrna came to the mental health clinic claiming she was pregnant. She said she had been raped by her caseworker when they went "to look at her land." Myrna reported that he injected her with a yellow liquid, whereupon she lost consciousness. On physical examination she was declared to be in good health but had gained ten pounds in three months. Her stomach was growing.
>
> Myrna often felt scared, cried a great deal, and needed company. She had had many fantasies about brides and weddings. Although she had been married for over thirty years, she now claimed she had never had sexual relations with her husband because he was physically incapacitated.

We found the discussion between the Spiritists and Myrna's therapist to be extremely interesting. The Spiritists diagnosed Myrna as "obsessed" because she wanted to have sex and children. This was "suggested to her mind" by a spirit and was a possible result of a spiritual debt. Her husband wasn't *spiritually* incapacitated and went into space (after he died) with the idea of having sexual relations with his wife; now she "calls" him in her loneliness. The social worker *had* violated her, although in another existence. Moreover, the Spiritists asserted that spirits can have sexual relations with living beings.

From her narrative it seemed that Myrna's therapist actually treated her condition as if it were believable. She talked with the caseworker, who admitted that he was afraid of Myrna. She also asked her patient about her sexual "fantasies." A psychiatrist at the case discussion session recommended that Myrna be told directly and strongly that she was not pregnant. Other Spiritists disagreed with the belief that an incarnated spirit, for example, Myrna's husband, decides what will happen in his or her life prior to incarnation. Their objection was based on the view that if this notion were true, the psychological cure of an individual would be impeded because there would be no possibility of change. One therapist did agree, however, that spirit-human sexual relations might be possible.

In summary, we heard both types of healers more or less agree that inner wishes could be physically expressed as actual symptoms or conditions, but they clearly disagreed as to the causes and dynamics of such symptoms. The Spiritist healers interpreted Myrna's condition as "real" but related to experience with spirits, but the therapists did not interpret beyond the notion of "fantasies" and applied their view of reality as that which can be seen and verified. The Spiritists' views were also prognostic; they asserted that Myrna's body was weak and that her tired spirit wanted to separate itself from its material existence. They explained that the intensity and intimacy of her dead husband's spirit predicted her own "passing over."

Another case of what could be labeled "conversion disorder" is interesting for the "miraculous cure" claimed by the Spiritist who saw the client after she had been to see medical doctors many times. No one seemed to be able to sort out the reason for the cure, not even the doctors who saw this young girl and, later, her father. From a medical perspective, the problem was diagnosed as being self-limited; from a Spiritist perspective, spirits attached-themselves to this family because of the father's failing to heed the call to work as a medium.

María

> Thirteen years of age, the oldest of two children, María suffered from painful red sores on her feet that turned into "burns," and the skin began to crack. She was in so much pain that she could hardly walk or sleep and was unable to attend school most of the time. Over three years, her mother took her to various clinics and finally to an allergist. However, the condition only seemed to worsen. Strangely, María's father began to have the same rash all over his body; his feet became bloody. At that point Doña Ana was recommended by a friend. Although María's mother was confirmed in her Catholicism, she felt she had to find a cure for her daughter and called this woman to her house.

María herself reported that Doña Ana "touched my feet and looked at my hands. She asked how I was and if I was in a lot of pain, and I said, 'Yes.' She then said that she would fight for me and put me into her prayers for six months. She said that I should be brought to the temple [*centro*] in order to improve. There she gave me *despojos* with water and oil and prayed in the name of Saint Lazarus."

In following María, we found that in three months she had improved so much that, according to her mother's report, she could wear shoes and was able to return to school. Her father also went to the temple and was cured. The only reason given by the healer for the illnesses was that the father had faculties but did not practice as a medium. In other words, his lack of interaction with the spirit world caused his problems to be visited upon his daughter. Once she was cured, then he received the spirit impact and became ill. Doña Ana described how the father began to be "neurotic" and came to the temple as well. There the "cause" was discovered.

We reflected upon the fact that although much about the father-daughter relationship was implied in the account of María's illness, it was never directly mentioned as related to the illness. Usually such matters are dealt with metaphorically through images of spirits who impact upon the bodies of clients and are sometimes even directly discussed. It seems that in this case, the only spiritual message was that the father was neglecting his responsibilities as a "developed" person, which implies that he was attending more to "dark," negatively valued matters than to working with "spirits of light." We had observed that Spiritist healers frequently do not bring the inner dynamics of interpersonal conflict to the surface. With this kind of problem, it is as if its cause is so hidden from the awareness of their clients that the healers do not want to bring it up, even metaphorically.

Conclusions and Observations on Bodily Distress

In this chapter I have presented information on some common attitudes and behavior in relation to the "body" among women in Puerto Rico and have shown that these notions and feelings have an edge that opens onto both distress about life events and circumstances and opportunities for communicating this distress by using the body as an idiomatic source of expression. I have also discussed cases of illness in which the body is the central focus of complaints, used in distinct ways for different types of disorders. In only one category of cases, those labeled here as "no psychiatric diagnosis," does the communication of bodily pain and malaise seem to refer directly to a physical dimension of experience, without complex elaboration along social, interpersonal, or moral dimensions. Yet even here distress generated in interpersonal relations forms a significant backdrop for much physical illness and can, for example, determine when the complaints will lead to a visit to a clinic or a healer.

Considering these data on the causes and experience of illness and its treatment, especially with regard to cases seen by the Spiritist healers, I cannot but agree with Kirmayer (1987:133; see also Kirmayer, 1984a) that "somatization," instead of being analysed as a psychological mechanism, is best explained in Puerto Rico through an analysis of "sociomatics," that is, the links between "social and somatic events." However, with regard to certain psychiatrically defined illnesses, such as "somatization disorders," even the Spiritist healers seem to recognize that some clients substitute body complaints for emotional states, as in the case of Lola.

I suggest that the key to understanding the body as a vehicle for expressions about illness causality among Hispanic peoples is that somatic symptoms are *meant* to direct attention to both specific types of psychosocial problems and patterned emotional responses. In a metaphoric way, bodily symptoms map distress. The complaint of *nervios*, as discussed by Low (1981, 1985) and others (Guarnaccia et al., 1989), is not to be taken at its face value as a physical symptom but is presented to the general medical practitioner as a signpost that other somatic complaints that accompany it can be referred to family conflict and to reproductive and sexual problems. Similarly, Tousignant's (1985) analysis of illness in Ecuador suggests that discourse on *pena* refers to biological symbols that echo psychological experience, which, rather than masking social conflict related to illness, directs attention to it. In these examples, it seems clear that the body is used as a code that keys aspects of the underlying cause and context of both somatic and psychological complaints.

In many of the cases described, the Spiritist healers said they "saw" (and felt) the physical complaint, which validated it for the client. But the complaint was then treated as a sign that opened onto evidence of spirit-person conflicts. It is this second step that goes beyond the physical dimension into the interpersonal-spiritual sphere that is so different from medical treatment. Doctors in Puerto Rico generally validate physical symptoms through laboratory tests but discount them as unimportant if tests do not confirm that they are signs of a defined disease syndrome. Doctors usually take somatic symptoms literally or may think of them as "somatization." For some illness syndromes, they inquire about stress at home or at work but rarely incorporate this information into an explanation of the cause of the illness or into a focus of treatment. Body complaints are dealt with in yet a different way by mental health professionals, who search behind them for an emotionally disordered state, such as depression or anxiety, that they may represent. They pay attention to and treat disorder in a client's immediate social world but rarely touch upon deep, existential concerns or guilt over moral transgressions. Mental health workers most often seem to negate a client's experience of his or her body. In my opinion, this approach ignores the usefulness of this experience in Puerto Rican culture as a map and guide to what the sufferer may identify as his or her major source of distress, centered in the relationship between feelings about the self and interpersonal experience.

Given the examples of how women present their bodies to doctors, mental health professionals, and Spiritist mediums and how each type of healer uses different expressions of malaise to construct a diagnosis ("this is what is wrong") and a treatment plan, it seems that each type of healer is attacking the proverbial blind man's elephant from a different angle. Each can find patients and clients who respond positively to their concepts and methods and others who go on to look for relief elsewhere. There are also those who rotate among all of the possible sources of help.

Notes

1. In this regard, Mechanic (1972:1135) notes how feelings about one's strength are threatened by a "near miss," which can "dramatically undermine one's sense of invulnerability and may lead to extreme anxiety and fear reactions."

2. Kirmayer (1986) points out that clinicians readily make organic versus psychological causal decisions prior to making a diagnosis. Once they find one or the other in evidence, they often rule out a multicausal explanation. The therapists seeing María seem to have operated in just this way.

3. Rivera Ramos (1985) echoes this view with regard to both menopause and sterilization.

11

Approaching the Self Through Illness and Healing

In order to function positively, the medial woman must have a strong ego vessel, one which knows its boundaries, can discriminate the personal from the transpersonal and can communicate. Her ego must also be permeable, so that she can receive the collective impressions which it is her task to mediate.

The medial woman's ego needs to be flexible, embodied and syntonic with the Feminine Self.

—Laurie Layton Schapira, *The Cassandra Complex*

Culture is not indigenous clothing that covers the universal human; it infuses individuals, fundamentally shaping and forming them and how they conceive of themselves and the world.

—Philip Cushman, "Why the Self is Empty"

In this book I describe a kaleidoscope of experiences of healing and suffering, especially of emotional distress and mental illness as expressed and observed by women in Puerto Rico. I have examined these experiences as events within two quite different healing systems. Women as healers—doctors and mental health professionals and Spiritists—assist in shaping their patients' interpretations of the causes, labels, and outcomes of their disorders (as do men as healers). I explore the discourse of women as healers and patients in order to arrive at patterned descriptions of suffering as well as analyses of its genesis and affective expression and its effect on interpersonal realms of experience.

As Harwood (1988) insightfully points out, the term "discourse" can be used in two ways: it can label the dialogue or conversations between two or more individuals, particularly when they have differing perspectives, or it can refer to the concepts, values, and symbols of a particular group. In this book I have used discourse in both ways: in the first way to describe how distress manifests in women and how it is thought about and *felt* by people with differing views of the healing task. But I have also used discourse to develop interpretations and explanations about particular genres of distress. This latter task represents the pursuit of meaning by healers and patients as both a collective venture and an important personal need. I assume that this pursuit is shared by people like myself (and you, the reader) who are clinicians, social scientists, and human beings vitally interested in learning about and helping women in distress.

Some researchers suggest that the pursuit of meaning is the most important function of healers (Frank, 1961; Frank et al., 1978; Kleinman and Sung, 1979; Kleinman, 1988; Fuller Torrey, 1986; Finkler, 1985) because the sufferer is helped to redefine her relationship to her complaints as well as the complaints themselves and can become hopeful of relief or accept experiences of distress as characteristics of her self. And even if complaints remain after treatment or healing, the sufferer may be able to make social or behavioral gains over conditions and circumstances that formerly impeded her. This observation points to an important goal of the descriptions of the experiences of Puerto Rican women: an exploration of the interface between an individual's response to malaise and the processes by which the culture patterns the experience of suffering, thus rendering it meaningful and malleable, open to treatment and change.

Although psychiatric and medical concepts (and categories) of disease represent only one of the paradigms that shape illness experience in Puerto Rico, in this book I have used them as a template against which to compare nonmedical—that is, idiosyncratic and Spiritist—paradigms and explanations. The same woman, during one episode of illness, may experience "depression" in terms of hallucinations, poor or excessive appetite, memory problems, and feelings of sadness or depression, if she presents to a mental health clinic; or, alternatively, in terms of "backaches," "legaches," and "fear," if she attends a Spiritist session. However, she will probably experience "headaches," "sleep disturbances," and "nervousness" regardless of the resource she uses. If we encounter her at the mental health clinic, she may explain her distress as due to disordered or out-of-control mind, behavior, or lifestyle. In the Spiritist session she will probably have her distress explained as an "obsession." And if we encounter her before she seeks help from either of these treatment resources, she may describe her problems as due to difficulties with her husband or children (or to their having abandoned her).

To answer questions about whether one type of treatment is more effective than another, we have to underscore the observation we make in this book that healing traditions within the same society, as in Puerto Rico, can differ radically in their views about what constitutes treatment in general and "good" treatment in particular. Moreover, the values and concepts used to assess treatment outcome are usually not the same for patients and healers. As an example, if we compare the psychiatric treatment of a woman suffering from dysthymic disorder with the Spiritist treatment of a woman suffering from a statistically equivalent complaint profile, we see that some goals of these very different treatments are shared. These goals are the elimination of sleep problems, the elevation of depressed mood, the lessening of agitation and anxiety or nervousness, and the alleviation or adjustment of marital and family problems. But other goals of these differing treatments are far from commensurate, such as Spiritists' insistence that for some "depressed/obsessed" women, a cure depends upon their submitting to a process of personal transformation and becoming healers. And for most women, according to Spiritists, a cure cannot be achieved without some discovery about their selves and the meanings their lives hold. In Spiritist practice, "cure" as a concept is not meaningful; the word "*sanar*" (to heal, make whole) is most frequently used. "Healing" means accepting and living with wounds as well as changing the perceptions of distress.

This discussion highlights the fact that all systems of intervention in emotional distress and disorder can potentially help in positive ways (although not in all cases at all times), albeit in different ways. A common element in this help is the restructuring of the assumptive world of the sufferer through communications about healthy and pain-relieving meanings focused on the body, self, and world. However, some treatments may not be effective or may even be perceived as antitherapeutic, as in many of the case examples described earlier in this book.[1] We systematically observed that patients of therapists and clients of Spiritists in almost equal proportions got better, stayed the same, or felt that treatment had not been effective in relation to all types of complaints (Koss, 1987). Perhaps the important question is not about the outcome of healing interventions but about the experience of the process, as I have suggested throughout this book (see also Csordas, 1988). We have to note that the Spiritist healing process is largely incremental and open-ended; it is a life process with ongoing implications and effects, not a limited form of treatment for a single episode of distress labeled as "disease." Most psychiatric treatment shares these goals with Spiritism and intends (also hopes) to restore the disordered person to more adequate functioning and a satisfying life in the future. However, Spiritists go one step further. Their assumption and deep belief that healing is a route to the "evolution" of the self (*el ser propio*) and that its core process is personal transformation applies even to the client who is treated only once at a Spiritist session. And the developed healer fully intends to follow a sacred commitment to an existential relationship with all beings (spirits) associated with her self in past, present, and future lives.

It seems necessary to digress somewhat before launching into a discussion of women's psychology in Puerto Rico from the perspectives of suffering and healing. I have used the concept of "self" throughout in a way that follows an old perspective in anthropology and a more recent one in psychology—that of the "culturally constituted self" (Hallowell, 1955; Geertz, 1973;

Cushman, 1990). Most Western psychologies treat the "self" as a universal, unitary structure, although they agree that its content contains infinite, individual variations. Only in the last decade have cogent discussions appeared about indigenous psychologies and how other cultures construct notions about the nature of the self in specific ways (Heelas and Lock, 1981; Sampson, 1988). The "self" without its Western psychological trappings is simply a concept of the person as human, defined by the traditions and shared understandings of a particular cultural group and imparted to all neonates in that group so that each person forms within himself or herself notions and images of who they are within the limits of their culture's template for human being. The individual's unique set of experiences determines how his or her notions of self fit within that general template. Culturally patterned therapies intend to assist and bring about change when individuals' self-concepts do not fit well enough to afford a level of comfort in terms of inner peace and outer harmony. It is in this sense that all types of healers in this study "work" with women who suffer emotional and cognitive distress (though to different extents); some women become healers themselves when they seek self-change.

Both psychological and traditional healers intend to work with elements of self beyond those that are conscious and visible, beyond verbal expressions and behavior: psychiatrists use "psyche" or "personality," psychoanalysts use the "unconscious" (as referred to in the quotation from Schapira in the epigraph at the beginning of this chapter, in which self includes both conscious and unconscious dimensions), and Spiritists work with "spirits." All of these are culturally constituted constructs about human "being" that structure individuals' awareness about themselves. In this chapter I propose that "healing" (in whatever form) reconstitutes the self in particular ways. I focus on the way healing affects the gendered self, the awareness of the feminine. Thus if one suffers and undertakes therapy or undergoes healing, emotional distress can be said to be "self"-seeking.

Psychology of Women in Puerto Rico: Medial Women

Women as healers are "medial women" immersed in the "psychic atmosphere of their environment and the spirit of their period" (Wolff, 1956). Although the mental health professionals and doctors in this study were not as directly in touch with the nether regions of the self (the psyche, the unconscious, or "spirit" images) as were the Spiritists, they too relied upon internal messages when treating other women (or men). This might not be obvious when a doctor prescribes medication for an infection or a tranquilizer for nervousness but *is* present when the doctor empathically inquires into the troubled atmosphere of the patient's family life or attempts to explore her uncomfortable feelings toward her body. Women as healers are genuinely concerned with how women can survive in a social environment that is unstable and uncertain for both sexes but that distinctly favors men. Personal mediation of distress is rarely taught in medical schools and is only sometimes (in some places) a part of the training of psychologists and social workers (Konner, 1987). However, all of the women healers in this book appeared to be well disposed toward employing their medial faculties in their healing work. But they were also at the forefront of women in Puerto Rico who sought autonomy and self-fulfillment; therefore they commonly examined the circumstances that influenced their patients' disorders and felt them to be kin to their own needs and distress.

As described in Chapter 5, the old values and regimens of male authoritarianism persist (although they are less evident in public spheres) despite the essential participation of women in the work force and despite the fact that a few women have now been appointed or elected to important political and social positions. This is "social progress" resulting from an industrialized and touristic economy. However, it does not reach far down into women's lives, nor does it have much effect on women in the lowest socioeconomic classes. A column written by an important, upper-class woman (Benitez, 1987) reports that ten years ago the then newly formed Committee on Women's Rights noted that despite better education, a woman had only a "minimal part of a man's opportunities to occupy positions of leadership in government service, and even fewer opportunities in the private sector." Although this is less true today, it is still an overwhelming fact; most women in Puerto Rico can hardly aspire to positions that might give them a tenth of the power and money held by men. The underside of all this is that even middle-class women are as bound to their homes and families as ever. If they work outside, job satisfaction is almost always less than that of male peers because women's priority is still the sacred job of homemaker—even if they spend fewer hours at home than at the workplace. As described earlier, most of a woman's sense of self-worth comes from marital and familial relationships. To say that these roles are a primary source of stress resulting in greater negativism toward their marriages and resentment and ambivalence toward their families, as does Richman (1984), is accurate. However, it is grossly understated when applied to lower-class women because their dependency upon home-centered roles is increasingly affected by familial dysfunction expressed as domestic violence, incest, and abandonment, unrelieved in the case of women who lack education and job skills. Middle-class women may not suffer as much from violence, but they do suffer the abandonment and also the stress that accompanies their tremendous efforts to do it all—homemaking, superlative mothering, and working in a rewarding career.

I observe such "truths" in order to deflect the view that only women who are patients or clients of therapists, doctors, and healers are stressed by the patterns of their lives in Puerto Rico. It is just that some women are less able to cope with their distress, either in quiet, muted ways or by becoming healers or superwoman professionals. It would seem that women as patients lack strong selves that would allow them to separate the personal from the cultural circumstances in which they find themselves. Unlike healers, they have not developed medial faculties that can receive and process the pain and slights they so acutely feel and then return them to the world in a transformed and useful form. Instead, women as patients accept and even collude in an ethos of feminine dependency that preempts an inner attitude of autonomy.

A case described by a Spiritist medium at a Project case review session images feelings of dependency and deep anxiety associated with being unable to take control of one's life. The case illustrates that these feelings and attitudes are passed on from mothers to daughters in an endless cycle. Doña Elisa reported:

> There are three victims of these problems. One is the grandmother of the girl, who is seventeen years old [the identified target of spirit attack]. The three are women: a girl, her mother, and grandmother. In the last months they all suffered certain strange symptoms: crying spells, intranquility, and agitation. And all three had fractured a leg, although under different circumstances. They had seen doctors, psychologists, and psychiatrists for those symptoms they had, that depression. A Spiritist had actually predicted the leg fractures in their futures [and then they occurred]. A group of us went to their home. The *videncias* began. I saw a narrow street full of stone houses. All this passed through my mind. That is called *plasmación*, not *videncia*, because it's like a movie that gives all the details. Then in this small street, similar to Old San Juan but more like Europe, there was suddenly a door. As I looked in, someone hit a man, and he fell to the floor face up. I saw that he had a knife in his back. It was like a common *cantina*, I imagine, like the Middle Ages. Another body was on a table in front of a man with a wooden leg, without teeth, ugly, bearded, and laughing. He had just killed that humpbacked person on the table. Still another man was there and he was big and strong and could have prevented the two deaths but did nothing.
>
> A medium at the gathering then took [was possessed by] the spirit of the hunchbacked man, who had gone into the *cantina* to ask for food and was then killed. The spirit harbored great anger against the three men—against the one who killed him and the others who witnessed it. The three women then told about everything that was happening to them, and I felt a tremendous head pain as if I had been hit. I then told them my impression that the man who killed the hunchback was [incarnated in] the girl. The spirit of the hunchback had been seeking revenge on the girl and on her mother and grandmother with a "mania" to break their legs so they would be deformed like he was.

This spirit "evidence" metaphorically but vividly illustrates feelings of helplessness that women pass on to their daughters. These feelings are often imaged as pursuit by an evil man with intent to harm. In my interpretation, this image illustrates women's shared guilt over a barely conscious sense that they possess crippling inner "killers" with deformed natures. If we were to look at it from an analytic perspective, we might say that they are expressing the feeling that the deformed, very vulnerable hunchback aspect of their selves is an eternal inner possibility. From a psychological perspective, we might appreciate that some women exhibit fears of, or actual vulnerability to, injury that makes it difficult for them to function (that is, walk) in the world.

This case presentation images the feelings that women as patients have in relation to their inability to control their lives, a condition sometimes described as "hysteria" in early psychiatric writings and linked to anxiety disorders in later ones. (See Cixous and Clement, 1986, and Schapira, 1988.) However (as amply illustrated throughout this book), in my observations, emotional distress can also be simultaneously experienced as a challenge through which to discover the true nature of one's self as a complex composite of many personalities, some of which are dark and destructive but also possessed of considerable strength and power.

Boddy (1988:19), describing possession-illness in Northern Sudanese women, says that it "enables a woman to evolve" by providing her with experiences of her "non-self" and thus "enhancing her sense of personhood." As I have described in Chapters 3 and 4, this is certainly the case with regard to Spiritist healers. They acquire their personal spirit guides through possession states that originate in illness and severe emotional distress. Their clients, although diagnosed as plagued by molesting spirit presences, do not usually become possessed. However, along with patients of doctors and mental health professionals, they are forced to become familiar with the darker, devil-like sides of their beings through experiencing their bodies and spirits as having turned against them. Deep within the tragedy of the inability to exorcise, or even separate one's self from, the diabolic tortures of deep emotional disorder, patients and clients come to glimpse seeds of change and self-transcendence—especially if guided to do so. And some experiences of suffering even seem to spontaneously produce positive attitudes toward acquiring self-knowledge.

Unfortunately, most psychiatric, psychological, and medical treatment modalities do not explicitly include a positive perspective on emotional disorder as illness, in contrast to Spiritism. And, of course, Spiritism does not always do what it intends for women (or men) as clients. As a healing system it both suffers and benefits from the absence of codification and standardization. In contrast to psychiatric and medical practices, much more is left to the inspiration of individual healers, who, lacking a standardized code of ethics, are then suspected of using their powers toward harmful ends when competition and jealousies arise (Koss, 1977; see also Faust, 1988).

Women are socially "medial" in Puerto Rican society in that they are perceived as being closer to the instinctual dimension of human being, largely because of their reproductive and mothering functions but, in my observation, also because they are perceived as central to everyone's else's well-being. Most important, women are seen as mediating between life and death in physical, psychological, and symbolic ways. This tends to bring about a focus on women (rather than men) as healers, even though some (though many fewer) men also display medial faculties. As already described in Chapter 5, the instinctual, animal side of human being is experienced as powerful, black, and potentially destructive, just as magic is categorized into both black and white practices and spirits are malevolent and benevolent (as well as "in between"). Paradoxically, acting through one's instincts is also felt to be desirable, but at the same time it is dangerous, or at the least, embarrassing. Thus it follows that the most popular spirit guide of women Spiritists is imaged as a black-skinned, strong, matronly woman—an obeah worker, the *madama*. She is a "dark feminine" image, the chthonic aspect of Woman.

Many social symbols illuminate women as sacred guardians of reproductive and regenerative pathways to the continuation of society. This is what informs and affirms a sense of personal continuity in everyone, men and women, and provides hope and succor when that continuity is threatened by severe malaise or illness. However, women are also perceived as failing miserably in carrying out the sacred aspects of their roles. (After all, isn't it more than men and children have a right to expect?) From the male perspective (with women often colluding), there are really only two kinds of women: those who succeed and those who fail—virgin mothers and whores. Because women as healers preside over life and death matters, they especially fall heir to these polar ways of apprehending women.

All of the foregoing can be related to a "Cassandra complex," which is the reluctance of men (and many women) to believe in the fundamental rationality of women's special capacity to see into worlds beyond the visible and the sensate (Schapira, 1988). The reader will recall that Cassandra predicted the conquest of Troy but was ignored. Just like the Trojan men of Cassandra's time, most Puerto Rican men feel uncomfortable if women have important roles in the big events of their society, the world, or the cosmos. (In my view, the famous late and only mayoress of San Juan gained her considerable stature largely by appearing to be like every man's mother, while behaving in astute, political ways.) Women who use their medial faculties are often labeled "hysterical" or evil, with all the ambivalence that misunderstood power attracts. This obtains because women in Puerto Rico, as elsewhere, are perceived as "acquiring their social identities and personal individuality solely in the sphere of the private," while men's personal identities are an amalgam of private and public aspects (Blair, 1981:212; see Koss, 1977). At the same time, healer women, even if their medial faculties remain covert or implicit in their work (as is the case of most women doctors, nurses, and psychologists), seek to expand their own psychological space beyond the private sphere and covertly guide their patients along this way. Even if this is not made explicit in their healing rites or clinical encounters, it is done implicitly through the dynamics of transference and countertransference in the therapeutic relationship. Moreover, they not only work to change or heal their own bodies and behavior but, as they described in indirect ways, they simultaneously work on their souls while working on others. Viewed in this way, healing is "self" work.

As Scarry (1985) so well illustrates, exploration and experience of pain are the "making and unmaking of the world" from the perspective of the sufferer. And by analogy, if illness, disability, and emotional disorder in their arbitrariness and surprise deconstruct the world of the patient by unmaking it, then healing is a way of remaking the world (Scheper-Hughes and Lock, 1987). The healing process can also remake and renew relationships with intimate, significant others; connection within "being" (as well as between beings) is a basic support for the feminine self (see Gilligan, 1982, and Ulanov, 1981).

In the zar cults in Ethiopia many ill women are believed to be possessed by zar spirits. Boddy (1988:19) identifies this interpretation of illness as an opportunity for the possessed woman to evolve, in much the same way that I have described the "development" of the medium-healer in Chapter 3. Boddy describes how the "existence of her non-self becomes subjectively real" to the possessed woman, who enters trance in order to come to terms with the spirit affecting her health. Although Spiritist clients are always potentially mediums-in-the-making (over one-third are diagnosed as in "development," but not all undergo it), they are thought to have been penetrated by illness- or problem-causing spirits. They, too, enter into confrontations and dialogues with the spirits causing them malaise; but unlike the spirits that medium-healers come to recognize as *guías* (amplifications of their panels of conscious selves), the *causa* spirits are exhorted to leave the clients. However, emotional disorder and severe problems are also opportunities to see one's life in a different light; the *causa* spirits are mirror images of the dark, negative side of one's self (as perhaps part-selves), as contrasted with the *guías*, who support and help both healers and patients. Although therapists' patients do not have these spirit mirrors for their therapies, they commonly reflect on interior issues of guilt and shame, moral dimensions of etiological notions about suffering that pervade Puerto Rican thought.

Conclusion

Illness can be thought of as a muted state of being, a lapse into a state of passivity much greater than one would normally experience. However, as I described earlier in relation to healer initiatory experiences, knowledge of spirits can be a source of expansion of the self, a way to connect one's idiosyncratic uniqueness to all of the possible others that make up our complex world of what I believe (with the Spiritists) to be multidimensional selves and their relationships.[2] Possession-trance is characterized by a sense of timelessness; through it, whether as the one possessed or as a dependent observer in search of relief or new information, one can come into contact with the cosmic whole and transcend the recurring feelings of aloneness and difference that emotional disorder as illness generally exacerbates.

The reader might now be thinking that this is all well and good for clients of the *Espiritistas*, but what about the others who see mental health professionals or medical doctors to heal their emotional disorders? Do they, too, find a way to transcend loneliness and an opportunity to expand their selves? Although notions about the evolution of one's spirit and the realization of one's soul through suffering are not formalized as aspects of psychological or medical treatments, a patient does enter into a state of communality within the world of suffering and particularly in relation to the therapist/doctor/healer who shapes and guides this world. These personal connections are vitalized through deeply shared understandings about death and shared visions of eternal life, which usually exist on an ideal plane for medical doctors and mental health workers. These ideals only partly differ from Spiritist beliefs about death and reincarnation of the spirit. In experiencing suffering and seeking healing, privacy is no longer possible. Although illness and emotional disorder may mute the social self and prevent the sufferer from asserting her autonomy and individual rights, they can also amplify that part of the self that shares its experience of being with other beings. Hillman (1975:71), referring to Freud and Jung and their patients, asserts that "symptoms, not therapists led this century to the soul. Their movement through pathology into soul is an experience repeated in each of us. We owe them much but we owe our pathologizing more."

All healers deal with the communal infinite in some sense, because healing and death are close companions. Healing is not simply an interpersonal process but is a "mode of immortality." It can lead to "communal resymbolization," as it often does for Spiritists and potentially can for all healers who hope to live on through their works (Lifton, 1970). Through healing acts, a moral sense of daily person-to-person responsibility is renewed. The central thesis of this book is that Puerto Rican women, as healers, often recognize and participate in these essential acts of renewal because they are prepared to do so by cultural understandings and expectations regarding their roles and behavior. Puerto Rican culture orients women toward pain, suffering, and caring for others.

Notes

1. At this point the reader may feel compelled to ask whether one of these healing systems is more effective than another as a source of help, especially in relation to a

particular illness or a particular type of emotional distress. One might also ask why we have portrayed Spiritist healing and beliefs in more detail than the other healing systems. Does that mean that they are superior? Assessing the effectiveness of treatments of illness across alternative healing systems is a difficult undertaking. The question of how to measure effectivity and outcomes is fraught with complexities yet to be fully sorted out (Kleinman and Sung, 1979). What constitutes "cure" and whether cure is actually a goal of treatment varies across healing systems in direct relation to differing concepts about the body: whether body and mind are considered separate or not, whether there is a concept of "mind," according to particular values attached to varying types of behavior and differently defined feeling states, and whether "spirit" or "soul" is implicated in illness and distress (and there are many other variables as well).

Few studies have compared outcomes of healing across systems because of these and a host of other difficulties. Finkler (1985) points out that effectivity in biomedicine is measured by the capacity of a practitioner to alter what is viewed as the natural history of a disease. Medical doctors are taught that they can remove or eliminate single causes of particular genres of distress, classified as "disease." In contrast, psychiatrists are more accustomed to the idea that all they can usually do is ameliorate noxious factors (both inner and outer) producing distress; but they also attempt to strengthen or change a patient's capacity to cope with life in a more orderly, satisfying fashion. One must note that the new disease load of chronic ailments is now being approached by medical doctors in a similar fashion.

In a substudy of the Project, I asked one hundred new patients and clients to rank the degree to which they expected help for each complaint. When treatment for that episode of illness was complete, I then asked these same people what they felt had occurred in relation to each complaint. I focused only on complaints, not on illness or disease labels. I found that therapists and Spiritists were treating just about the same types of complaints, although patients brought significantly more feeling complaints to therapists. However, Spiritist clients had a tendency to report higher expectations regarding treatment of all types of complaints, but especially of mood and feeling complaints. The most interesting finding of this small substudy was that although Spiritists' clients reported significantly higher satisfaction for treatment of mood and feeling complaints, therapists' patients rated therapists as better in treating thought complaints. This agrees with observations presented earlier that women suffering from psychoses are more likely to see mental health professionals, especially in the acute phases of their illness. Most important, comparison of differences between expectations and outcomes across the two healing systems showed that both patients and clients improved, stayed the same or worsened to almost exactly the same extent. This substudy of outcomes demonstrated no clear-cut division of labor between Spiritism and mental health care but only complementarity in relation to particular problems—such as the social and emotional support that Spiritists frequently provide for people with long-term mental or chronic illness in treatment at mental health or medical clinics. Moreover, approximately half of Spiritists' clients would not be diagnosed as psychiatrically ill, and thus the mediums provide care in the community to women who would be unlikely to receive other kinds of help.

Finkler (1985) comments that the difficulty of defining appropriate objective criteria to measure outcomes of treatment intervention in nonmedical healing systems led her to examine only "patient perceived symptoms or target complaints." However, she used the Cornell Medical Index, a checklist of 194 symptoms, to measure complaints among her Mexican Spiritualist temple goers and regulars. Although I too used the Cornell Medical Index, I relied much more upon naturally occurring patients' descriptions of complaints in order to avoid the bias of the clinical constructs that underlie such assessments.

2. See Ewing, 1990, for a discussion from an anthropological perspective on the "illusion of wholeness" in self-concepts.

Appendix: Methodology

The Approach

In this study I have used data on patients' and clients' complaints (*quejas*) as windows onto women's experience of distress and as points of departure for examining individual and social meanings and interpretations of distress and illness. As pointed out by Kleinman and Good (1985), it is the study of emotional disorders that shows us that people are both connected to and affected by the social and cultural patterns and contingencies of their daily lives. The cases of 990 women—patients or clients of project participants who presented for help at primary care clinics, mental health clinics, or Spiritist *centros*—classified across healer samples and the lens provided by a psychiatric nosological paradigm were used to explore parallels and differences between medical and mental illness concepts and treatment and Spiritist beliefs and practices (which follow a very different nosological paradigm). I first used the largest sample of therapist cases (from the three opportunity samples described earlier—770 therapist cases) as an initial road map, based upon very general psychiatric and medical diagnostic perspectives. The 220 Spiritist cases in the largest sample were then statistically superimposed upon this map according to the patterning of grouped complaints, as will be described.

The quantitative method of analysis used six higher-rank psychiatric categories (major depression, dysthymia, schizophrenia, anxiety disorders, somatoform disorders, and personality disorders) and two residual categories (deferred psychiatric diagnosis and no psychiatric diagnosis). Although DSMII (APA, 1968) diagnoses were employed by the mental health clinicians at the time of the Therapist-Spiritist Training Project in Puerto Rico (1976–1979), these higher-rank categories have been updated to reflect changes in the current Diagnostic and Statistical Manual (DSMIIIR, APA, 1987). The method reclassified all of the DSMII diagnoses according to the changes in diagnostic classification published in the DSMIII (APA, 1980), and this was then subsequently updated to DSMIIIR categories and diagnoses.

In order to validate the diagnostic classifications, multivariate tests were carried out. They showed significant main effects between gender and diagnostic category as well as significant interactions between categories (Table A.2). For the most part, men and women in Puerto Rico, as patients in mental health and primary care settings, present different complaint profiles across these psychiatric and nonpsychiatric diagnostic categories of emotional distress. It must be emphasized, however, that these naturally occurring complaint profiles are not equivalent to the symptom lists found in psychiatric diagnostic manuals, such as DSMIIIR, as criteria for making a diagnosis. Rather, I worked backward from therapists' diagnoses to an examination of the most frequent complaints of their patients (taken from therapists' records and elicited from patients), whose individual diagnoses fell within one of the seven categories. (I did not include a discussion of the "personality disorders" category because there were not enough cases to account for variations in subcategories of personality disorders [such as "narcissistic personality disorder," "multiple personality disorder," and so on], and the cultural complexities of making this type of diagnosis demand a separate study.)

As we saw in the text, there is essentially no overlap between the types of diagnoses made by therapists (mental health clinicians or medical doctors) and those made by Spiritists. This is to be expected given the very different assumptions made by each type of healer with respect to their very different etiological explanations of emotional disorder and illness. However, particular complaints of Spiritist clients overlap considerably with those presented by clients of therapists. It was therefore decided to attempt to determine the extent to which clients of Spiritists reported patterns of complaints that would have led a therapist to diagnose that individual as suffering from a psychiatric disorder. The primary statistical tool used to accomplish this was discriminant analysis (Huberty, 1975, 1984).

Discriminant analysis examines all possible complaint profiles, defined in each case as a linear combination of the original variables submitted to the analysis. It selects among them that profile that maximally discriminates among various *a priori* groups. The degree of discrimination (differentiation) was measured by the univariate F-ratio for differences among the groups on that linear combination (profile) of complaints. Once this absolutely optimal DISCRIMINANT FUNCTION had been identified, a second, third, and so on, linear combination of the measures was identified, subject to the constraint that scores on each discriminant function be uncorrelated with scores on all preceding discriminant functions, up to a total of such profiles (number of groups minus 1), each identifying one dimension along which the groups differed from each other.

For present purposes, the *a priori* groups consisted of patients of therapists or medical personnel who received a diagnosis of one of the eight categories listed above (but only seven—personality disorders were excluded—are used in the descriptions in this book). The variables used in defining linear combinations were the seventy-three "new symptoms," a complaint list that resulted after first condensing 753 individual complaints and grouping them by similarity into 422 complaints. The "new symptom" list was then based on complaints that appeared more than ten times in the sample of 990 patients and clients. These data were then submitted to the SPSS-X program, DISCRIMINANT (SPSS-X, Inc., 1983). An initial run identified four statistically significant (and mutually uncorrelated) discriminant functions; therefore, a second run restricting the classification stage to these four functions was used to (1) classify the patients with known (psychiatric) diagnoses on the basis of their scores on the four functions in order to get an indication of how well this four-function-based classification corresponded to the known diagnoses, and (2) apply the same classification criteria to the Spiritists' clients' complaint patterns to identify those clients who probably would have been classified as having a particular diagnosis had they described their complaints to a therapist rather than a Spiritist.

The classification procedure involves computing the mean score on each of the four discriminant functions for each of the *a priori* groups and then comparing a given subject's score on those four discriminant functions to the patterns of mean scores for the *a priori* groups in order to determine which group's pattern of scores that individual subject most closely matches. (More specifically, the Euclidean distance from the subject's discriminant function scores and the mean degree of freedom scores for a particular group is computed as the square root of the sum of the four squared differences on the four discriminant functions, and the subject is then assigned to that group for which her Euclidean distance measure is smallest.) In the present case, because various diagnoses occurred with greatly different frequencies, this procedure was altered slightly by use of the PRIOR=SIZE subcommand so that a subject was classified into a relatively rare diagnostic category only if her Euclideam distance from that group was considerably smaller than her distance from a more common group.

For women patients, application of this classification procedure yielded 57.27 percent overall agreement with the known diagnoses; this percentage ranged from 0 percent correct classification of the "psychodepressed" patients (that is, those with major depression) to 92 percent correct classification of the patients given no psychiatric diagnoses (see Table A.3). Although we could have greater confidence in the classification of individual Spiritist clients had the overall percentage of correct classifications of therapist clients been even higher, that figure is nonetheless considerably above the chance level of 12.5 percent and represents highly significant differences among the *a priori* groups on the four discriminant functions. (The canonical correlation between diagnostic category and score on the discriminant function was .704 for the first discriminant function and .487, .344, and .355 for the second through fourth discriminant functions, $p < .001$ in the first three cases and $p < .05$ for the fourth discriminant function.)

TABLE A.1 Complaint Profiles by Diagnostic Category (in percent)

Therapist Cases		Spiritist Cases (Reclassified)	
Complaint	**Frequency**	**Complaint Frequency**	
O. No Psychiatric Diagnosis		O. No Psychiatric Diagnosis	
(Medical Cases)	n = 348		n = 104
Headaches	16.0	Headaches	20.0
Stomach problems	14.0	Family problems	14.0
Fever	11.5	Legaches	12.0
Throat problems	10.0	Fatigue	12.0
Dizzy spells	9.0	Backaches	8.0
Sleep disturbances	7.0	Stomach problems	8.0
Chest/heart problems	6.6	Marital problems	8.0
Leg/feet problems	6.0		
Fatigue	6.0		
Intranquility	6.0		
Hostility	5.7		
Hypertension	5.7		
Back problems	4.5		
Appetite change	3.0		
1. Major Depression	n = 11	1. Major Depression	
Crying jags	54.0	No cases classified	
Sleep disturbances	54.0		
Hallucinations and/or visual	45.0		
Headaches/head problems	36.0		
Nervousness	36.0		
Intranquility	36.0		
Feels depressed	27.0		
Bad humor	18.0		
2. Dysthymia	n = 131	2. Dysthymia	n = 17
Sleep disturbances	57.0	Crying jags	53.0
Crying jags	52.0	Fear	53.0
Headaches/head problems	40.0	Headaches	47.0
Intranquility	37.0	Nervousness	41.0
Nervousness	26.0	Backaches	29.0
Hallucinations	16.0	Insomnia	23.5
Hostility	16.0	Intranquility	23.5
Memory problems	16.0	Legaches	17.6
Chest/heart problems	10.6		
Suicidal intent	9.0		
Sadness	9.0		
Appetite change	6.8		
Bad humor	6.1		

TABLE A.1 (Continued)

Therapist Cases		Spiritist Cases (Reclassified)	
Complaint	**Frequency**	**Complaint**	**Frequency**
3. Schizophrenic Disorders	n = 53	3. Schizophrenic Disorders	n = 1
Sleep disturbances	56.0	Feels depressed	100.0
Hostility	47.0	Nervousness	100.0
Hallucinations	45.0	Family problems	100.0
Intranquility	38.0	Marital problems	100.0
Headaches/head problems	34.0		
Crying jags	26.0		
Nervousness	26.0		
Feels depressed	19.0		
4. Somatization Disorders	n = 13	4. Somatization Disorders	n = 16
Intranquility	61.5	Pain in eyes	69.0
Headaches/head problems	54.0	Fatigue	69.0
Sleep disturbances	46.0	Headaches	62.5
Nervousness	38.0	Nervousness	44.0
Chest pain	30.7	Chest problems	37.5
Memory problems	30.7	Memory problems	37.5
Crying jags	30.7	Intranquility	37.5
Hostility	30.7	Sleep disturbances	31.0
		Backaches	25.0
		Family problems	25.0
5. Anxiety Disorders	n = 108	5. Anxiety Disorders	n = 51
Sleep disturbances	46.0	"Mind disturbed, blank"	43.0
Intranquility	41.6	Headaches	39.0
Headaches/head problems	37.0	Intranquility	35.0
Nervousness	28.7	Nervousness	29.0
Crying jags	26.0	Fatigue	27.0
Hallucinations	15.7	Chest/heart problems	25.0
Trembling[a]	14.8	Family problems	20.0
Bad humor	9.0	Sleep disturbances	14.0
6. Personality Disorders	n = 15	6. Personality Disorders	n = 6
Sleep disturbances	53.0	Throat problems	50.0
Nervousness	33.0	Fatigue	50.0
Hostility	26.0	Sleep disturbances	50.0
Intranquility	26.0	Nervousness	50.0
Headaches	26.0	Family problems	33.3
Chest/heart complaints	26.0	Headaches	33.3
Marital problems	33.3		

TABLE A.1 (Continued)

Therapist Cases		Spiritist Cases (Reclassified)	
Complaint	**Frequency**	**Complaint Frequency**	
7. Deferred Diagnosis	n = 91	7. Deferred (equivalent)	n = 25
Sleep disturbances	40.6	Headaches	44.0
Headaches	29.6	Fatigue	32.0
Intranquility	26.0	Backaches	28.0
Crying jags	19.7	Memory problems	28.0
Nervousness	15.3	Nervousness	20.0
Frightened[a]	10.9	Family problems	20.0
Eyes/vision problems[a]	8.8		

[a] Complaints that appear in only one or two diagnostic categories; most are of low frequency in the total sample.

Source: Compiled by author

TABLE A.2 Significance Tests on Sex Distribution by Diagnostic Category

1. Mental Health Therapists Only

	F		M		N	Z on hypothesis that % F = 50% in population	X^2 test of difference: this and overall % F
No Psych. Diag.	66	(44.0%)	84	(66.0%)	150	-1.470	N.S.
Major Depression	9	(50.0%)	9	(50.0%)	18	0	N.S.
Dysthymia	126	(65.6%)	66	(34.4%)	192	4.330***	p < .001
Schizophrenia	51	(34.7%)	96	(65.3%)	147	-3.712***	p < .001
Somatization	13	(65.0%)	7	(35.0%)	20	1.342	N.S.
Anxiety	102	(57.6%)	75	(42.4%)	177	2.029*	N.S.
Personality	15	(50.0%)	15	(50.0%)	30	0	N.S.
Deferred Diag.	66	(52.0%)	61	(48.0%)	127	0.444	N.S.
Totals:	448	(52.0%)	413	(48.0%)	861		

Overall X^2 on difference in % F across diagnostic categories = 43.87 with 7 df, p < .001.

2. Mental Health Therapist and M.D. Cases Combined

	F		M		N	Z on hypothesis that % F = 50.0% in population	X^2test of difference: this and overall % F
No Psych. Diag.	348	(54.3%)	293	(45.7%)	641	2.172	N.S.
Major Depression	11	(55.0%)	9	(45.0%)	20	0.894	N.S.
Dysthymia	131	(64.9%)	71	(35.1%)	202	4.222*	p < .05
Schizophrenia	53	(35.1%)	98	(64.9%)	151	-3.662***	p < .001
Somatization	13	(65.0%)	7	(35.0%)	20	1.342	N.S.
Anxiety	108	(57.8%)	79	(42.2%)	187	2.121*	N.S.
Pesonality	15	(50.0%)	15	(50.0%)	30	0	N.S.
Deferred Diag.	91	(54.2%)	77	(45.8%)	168	1.080	N.S.
Totals:	770		649		1419		

Overall X^2 = 33.542 with 7 df, p < .001.

Source: Compiled by author

TABLE A.3 Differences Among Stepwise-Classified Therapists' and Spiritists' Patients

Classification Results for Therapists' Cases Selected for Use in the Analysis

		Predicted Group Membership							
Actual Group	**No. of Cases**	**0**	**1**	**2**	**3**	**4**	**5**	**6**	**7**
Group 0 None	348	288 82.8%	3 0.9%	9 2.6%	9 2.6%	5 1.4%	10 2.9%	5 1.4%	19 5.5%
Group 1 Psychodepressed	11	1 9.1%	6 54.5%	1 9.1%	1 9.1%	1 9.1%	0 0.0%	1 9.1%	0 0.0%
Group 2 Depressed	131	9 6.9%	13 9.9%	67 51.1%	7 5.3%	0 0.0%	16 12.2%	12 9.2%	7 5.3%
Group 3 Schizophrenic	53	4 7.5%	13 24.5%	4 7.5%	15 28.3%	4 7.5%	7 13.2%	2 3.8%	4 7.5%
Group 4 Somatic and Dissociative Disorder	13	0 0.0%	0 0.0%	2 15.4%	2 15.4%	7 53.8%	1 7.7%	0 0.0%	1 7.7%
Group 5 Anxiety Disorder	108	15 13.9%	4 3.7%	15 13.9%	10 9.3%	6 5.6%	46 42.6%	6 5.6%	6 5.6%
Group 6 Personality Disorder	15	1 6.7%	0 0.0%	3 20.0%	0 0.0%	1 6.7%	4 26.7%	4 26.7%	2 13.3%
Group 7 Deferred Diagnosis	91	35 38.5%	5 5.5%	16 17.6%	3 3.3%	5 5.5%	11 12.1%	8 8.8%	8 8.8%

Percent of "grouped" cases correctly classified: 57.27%

TABLE A.3 (Continued)

Classification Results for Spiritists' Cases Selected for Use in the Analysis

		Predicted Group Membership							
Actual Group	**No. of Cases**	**0**	**1**	**2**	**3**	**4**	**5**	**6**	**7**
Group 0 None	174	65 37.4%	0 0.0%	17 9.8%	1 0.6%	16 9.2%	49 28.2%	5 2.9%	21 12.1%
Group 1 Psychodepressed	0	0 0.0%	0 0.0%	0 0.0%	0 0.0%	0 0.0%	0 0.0%	0 0.0%	0 0.0%
Group 2 Depressed	0	0 0.0%	0 0.0%	0 0.0%	0 0.0%	0 0.0%	0 0.0%	0 0.0%	0 0.0%
Group 3 Schizophrenic	0	0 0.0%	0 0.0%	0 0.0%	0 0.0%	0 0.0%	0 0.0%	0 0.0%	0 0.0%
Group 4 Somatic and Dissociative Disorder	0	0 0.0%	0 0.0%	0 0.0%	0 0.0%	0 0.0%	0 0.0%	0 0.0%	0 0.0%
Group 5 Anxiety Disorder	0	0 0.0%	0 0.0%	0 0.0%	0 0.0%	0 0.0%	0 0.0%	0 0.0%	0 0.0%
Group 6 Personality Disorder	0	0 0.0%	0 0.0%	0 0.0%	0 0.0%	0 0.0%	0 0.0%	0 0.0%	0 0.0%
Group 7 Deferred Diagnosis	46	39 84.8%	0 0.0%	0 0.0%	0 0.0%	0 0.0%	2 4.3%	1 2.2%	4 8.7%

Percent of "grouped" cases correctly classified: 31.36%

Classification Processing Summary
990 cases were processed
0 cases were excluded for missing or out-of-range group codes
0 cases had at least one missing discriminating variable
990 cases were used for printed output
990 cases were written into the active file

Source: Compiled by author

TABLE A.4 Patient/Client Population by Age and Gender

Age F (%)	Therapist M (%)	F (%)	Spiritist M (%)	
1 - 11	2	2	-	-
12 - 18	2	9	2	2
19 - 30	4	15	20	19
31 - 55	22	26	22	15
56+	11	7	11	9
Totals:	41	59	55	45

Source: Compiled by author

TABLE A.5 Patient/Client Population by Occupation and Gender

	Therapist		Spiritist	
Occupation	F (%)	M (%)	F (%)	M (%)
Unknown	4	2	5	7
Student	2	11	6	7
Professional	2	2	2	2
White Collar[a]	2	-	9	7
Blue Collar[b]	2	22	7	11
Housewife	20	2	22	-
Unemployed/Retired	7	20	4	11
Child/Infant	2	-	-	-
Totals:	41	59	55	45

[a] Includes secretary, office clerk, store manager
[b] Includes seamstress, laborer, carpenter/mechanic, factory worker, engraver, cook

Source: Compiled by author

Bibliography

Abad, Vicente, and E. Boyce. 1979. "Issues in Psychiatric Evaluations of Puerto Ricans: A Socio-Cultural Perspective." *Journal of Operational Psychiatry* 10(1):28–39.

Acosta-Belen, Edna. 1980. Ideología e Imagenes de la Mujeres en la Literatura Puertorriqueña/Contempo. In *La Mujer en la Sociedad Puertorriqueña,* 125–156. Rio Piedras, Puerto Rico: Ediciones Huracan.

Acosta-Belen, Edna, and B. R. Sjostrom. 1980. La Mujer Puertorriqueña en la Fase Educativa y el Ejercicio Profesional. In *La Mujer en la Sociedad Puertorriqueña.* 109–124. Rio Piedras, Puerto Rico: Ediciones Huracan.

Al-Issa, I., ed. 1982. *The Psychopathology of Women.* Baltimore: Prentice Hall.

American Psychiatric Association. 1968. *Diagnostic and Statistical Manual of Mental Disorders.* 2d ed. Washington, D.C.

______. 1980. *Diagnostic and Statistical Manual of Mental Disorders.* 3d ed. Washington, D.C.

______. 1987. *Diagnostic and Statistical Manual of Mental Disorders.* 3d rev. ed. Washington, D.C.

Ardener, Shirley, ed. 1978. *Defining Females.* London: Crown Helm.

Barsky, A. J., and G. L. Klerman. 1983. "Overview: Hypochondriasis, Bodily Complaints and Somatic Styles." *American Journal of Psychiatry* 140(3):273–283.

Beck, A. T. 1976. *Cognitive Therapy and Emotional Disorders.* New York: International Universities Press.

Benitez, Celeste. 1987. "Woman's Week." *The San Juan Star,* Thursday, March 5.

Blair, Juliet. 1981. Private Parts in Public Places: The Case of Actresses. In S. Ardener, ed., *Woman and Space.* London: Croom Helm.

Boddy, Janice. 1988. "Spirits and Selves in Northern Sudan: The Cultural Therapies of Possession and Trance." *American Ethnologist* 15(1):4–27.

Borkovec, T. D. 1985. The Role of Cognitive and Somatic Cues in Anxiety and Anxiety Disorders: Worry and Relation Induced Anxiety. In H. A. Tuma and J. D. Maser, eds., *Anxiety and the Anxiety Disorders,* 463–478. New Jersey: Laurence Erlbaum Assoc.

Bourguignon, Erica. 1975. *Importante Papel de las Mujeres en los Cuentos Afroamericanos.* Caracas, Venezuela: Universidad Católica Andrés Bello, Instituto de Investigación Historica.

Bravo, Milagros, G. Canino, M. Rubio-Stipec, and M. Woodbury- Farina. 1991. "A Cross-Cultural Adaptation of a Psychiatric Epidemiologic Instrument: The Diagnostic Interview Schedule's Adaptation in Puerto Rico." *Culture, Medicine, and Psychiatry* 15(1):1–18.

Brody, Eugene B. 1973. *The Lost Ones: Social Forces and Mental Illness in Rio de Janeiro*. New York: International Universities Press.

Brown, George W., and T. Harris. 1978. *Social Origins of Depression*. New York: Free Press.

Canino, Glorisa. 1982. The Hispanic Woman: Sociocultural Influences on Diagnoses and Treatment. In R. M. Becerra, M. Karno, and J. Escobar, eds., *Mental Health and Hispanic Americans: Clinical Perspectives*, 117–138. New York: Grune and Stratton.

______. 1988. "Somatization and Somatization Disorders in Puerto Rico." Paper presented at the annual American Psychiatric Association Meeting, Montreal, Canada.

Canino, Glorisa, and Ian A. Canino. 1982. "Culturally Syntonic Family Therapy for Migrant Puerto Ricans." *Hospital and Community Psychiatry* 33:299–303.

Canino, Glorisa, H. Bird, P. Shrout, M. Rubio-Stipec, M. Bravo, R. Martinez, M. Sesman, A. Guzman, L. Guevara, and H. Costas. 1987a. "The Spanish Diagnostic Interview Schedule: Reliability and Concordance with Clinical Diagnoses in Puerto Rico." *Archives of General Psychiatry* 44:720–726.

Canino, G. J., H. Bird, P. Shrout, M. Rubio-Stipec, M. Bravo, R. Martinez, M. Sesman, and L. Guevara. 1987b. "The Prevalence of Specific Psychiatric Disorders in Puerto Rico." *Archives of General Psychiatry* 44:727–735.

Canino, Glorisa, M. Rubio-Stipec, P. Shrout, M. Bravo, R. Stolberg, and H. Bird. 1987c. "Sex Differences and Depression in Puerto Rico." *Psychology of Women Quarterly* 11:443–459.

Canino, Glorisa, J. Helzer, M. Rubio-Stipec, H. Bird, and M. Bravo. 1988. "A Cross-Cultural Analysis of Anxiety Disorders." Manuscript.

Carr, Raymond. 1985. *Puerto Rico: A Colonial Experiment*. New York: Vintage Books.

Chodorow, Nancy. 1978. *The Reproduction of Mothering*. Berkeley: University of California Press.

Christensen, Edward W. 1979. The Puerto Rican Woman: A Profile. In Edna Acosta-Belen, ed., *The Puerto Rican Woman*, 51–63. New York: Praeger.

Cixous, Helene, and Catherine Clement. 1986. *The Newly Born Woman*. Translated by Betsy Wing. Minneapolis: University of Minnesota Press.

Cohen, Lucy. 1979. *Culture, Disease and Stress Among Latino Immigrants*. Washington, D.C.: Smithsonian Institute, Research Institute on Immigration and Ethnic Studies.

Crapanzano, Vincent, and Vivian Garrison, eds. 1977. *Case Studies in Spirit Possession*. New York: John Wiley and Sons.

Csordas, Thomas J. 1988. "Elements of Charismatic Persuasion and Healing." *Medical Anthropology Quarterly* 2(2):121–142.

Cushman, Philip. 1990. "Why the Self is Empty: Toward a Historically Situated Psychology." *American Psychologist* 45:599–611.

Davis, D. L., and N. O. Whitten. 1988. "Medical and Popular Traditions of Nerves." *Social Science and Medicine* 26(12):1209–1221.

Davis, D. L., and P. J. Guarnaccia. 1989. "Introduction: Health, Culture and the Nature of Nerves." *Medical Anthropology* 11(1):1–14, special edition.

de Burgos, Julia. 1964. *Cuadernos de Poesia*. Vol. 9. San Juan, Puerto Rico: Instituto de Cultura.

Dobzhansky, Theodosius. 1975. Evolutionary Roots of Family Ethics and Group Ethics in the Centrality of Science and Absolute Values. In *Proceedings of the Fourth International Conference of the Unity of the Sciences,* 411–427. New York.

Dohrenwend, B. P. 1967. "Social Status, Stress and Physiological Problems." *American Journal of Public Health* 57(4):625–632.

Eichenbaum, Louise, and Susie Orbach. 1983a. *Understanding Women: A Feminist Psychoanalytic Approach.* New York: Basic Books.

______. 1983b. *What Do Women Want?* New York: Berkeley.

Eliade, Mircea. 1964. *Shamanism: Archaic Techniques of Ecstasy.* Princeton: Princeton University Press.

Ewing, Katherine. 1990. "The Illusion of Wholeness: Culture, Self, and the Experience of Inconsistency." *Ethos* 18:251–278.

Falloon, R. H., J. L. Boyd, C. W. McGill, J. S. Strang, and H. B. Moss. 1981. Family Management Training in the Community Care of Schizophrenia. In M. Goldstein, ed., *New Directions in Interviews with Families of Schizophrenics,* No. 12, 61–77. San Francisco: Jossey-Bass.

Farr, Robert M. 1981. On the Nature of Human Nature and the Science of Behavior. In Paul L. Heelas and Andrew J. Lock, eds., *Indigenous Psychologies: The Anthropology of the Self.* San Diego: Academic Press.

Faust, Betty B. 1988. When is a Midwife a Witch?: A Case Study from a Modernizing Maya Village. In P. Whelehan and contributors, eds., *Women and Health.* Massachusetts: Bergin and Garvey.

Fernández Marina, R. 1961. "The Puerto Rican Syndrome: Its Dynamics and Cultural Determinants." *Psychiatry* 24:79–82.

Fernández Marina, R., E. D. Maldonado Sierra, and R. D. Trend. 1958. "Three Basic Themes in Mexican and Puerto Rican Family Values." *Journal of Social Psychology* 48:167–181.

Finkler, Kaja. 1985. *Spiritualist Healers in Mexico.* New York: Bergin and Garvey.

Frank, Jerome D. 1961. *Persuasion and Healing.* Baltimore: Johns Hopkins.

Frank, Jerome D., R. Hoehn-Saric, S. D. Imber, et al. 1978. *Effective Ingredients of Successful Psychotherapy.* New York: Brunner Mazel.

Frerichs, Robert R., C. S. Aneshensel, and V. A. Clark. 1981. "Prevalence of Depression in Los Angeles County." *Journal of Epidemiology* 113:691–699.

Fuller Torrey, Edwin. 1986. *Witchdoctors and Psychiatrists.* rev. ed. New York: Harper and Row.

Gaines, Atwood, and P. Farmer. 1986. "Visible Saints: Social Cynosures and Dysphoria in the Mediterranean Tradition." *Culture, Medicine and Psychiatry* 10:295–330.

Ganellan, R. J., W. Matuzas, E. H. Uhlenhuth, R. Glass, and C. R. Easton. 1986. "Panic Disorder, Agoraphobia and Anxiety-Relevant Cognitive Style." *Journal of Affective Disorders* 11:219–225.

Garrison, Vivian. 1977a. "Doctor, Espiritista or Psychiatrist?: Health-Seeking Behavior in a Puerto Rican Neighborhood of New York City." *Medical Anthropology* 1:64–185.

______. 1977b. "The 'Puerto Rican Syndrome.'" In V. Crapanzano and V. Garrison, eds., *Espiritismo in Case Studies in Spirit Possession,* 383–449. New York: John Wiley and Sons.

______. 1978. "Support Systems of Schizophrenic and Nonschizophrenic Puerto Rican Women in New York City." *Schizophrenia Bulletin* 4:561–596.

______. 1979. "The Inner-City Support Systems Project: Adaptation of the Miami Model of Culturally Relevant Mental Health Care." Paper presented at the annual meeting of the Society for Applied Anthropology, Philadelphia, March 15–17.

Gaviria, Moises, and Ronald Wintrob. 1976. "Supernatural Influence in Psychopathology: Puerto Rican Folk Beliefs about Mental Illness." *Journal of the Canadian Psychiatric Association* 21:361–369.

Geertz, Clifford. 1973. Ritual and Social Change: A Javanese Example. In C. Geertz, ed., *The Interpretation of Cultures*, 142–169. New York: Basic Books.

Gilligan, Carol. 1982. *In a Different Voice*. Boston: Harvard University Press.

Good, Byron J., and M. J. Good. 1982. The Meaning of Symptoms: A Cultural Hermeneutic Model for Clinical Practice. In L. Eisenberg and A. Kleinman, eds., *The Relevance of Social Sciences for Medicine*. Dordrecht, Holland: D. Reidel Publishing Company.

Good, Byron J., and A. Kleinman. 1985. Culture and Anxiety: Cross-Cultural Evidence for the Patterning of Anxiety Disorders. In A. H. Tuma and J. Maser, eds., *Anxiety and the Anxiety Disorders*, 297–323. New Jersey: Laurence Erlbaum Assoc.

Good, J., M. Del Vecchio, and R. Manadi. 1985. The Interpretation of Iranian Depressive Illness and Dysphoric Affect. In A. Kleinman and B. Good, eds., *Culture and Depression*. Berkeley: University of California Press.

Gravas, T. 1986–1987. "*Maltrato* Fisico a la Mujer en Puerto Rico." *Homine* 10:197–200.

Groesbeck, C. Jess. 1975. "The Archetypal Image of the Wounded Healer." *Journal of Analytical Psychology* 20:122–145.

Guarnaccia, P., and P. Farias. 1988. "The Social Meanings of *Nervios*: A Case Study of a Central American Woman." *Social Science and Medicine* 26(12):1223–1231.

Guarnaccia, P. J., V. de la Cancela, and E. Carillo. 1989a. "The Multiple Meanings of *Ataques de Nervios*." *Medical Anthropology* 11(1):47–62, special edition, D. L. Davis and P. J. Guarnaccia, guest eds.

Guarnaccia, P. J., M. Rubio-Stipes, and G. Canino. 1989b. "*Ataques de Nervios* in the Puerto Rico Diagnostic Interview Schedule: The Impact of Cultural Categories on Psychiatric Epidemiology." *Culture, Medicine and Psychiatry* 13(3):275–295.

Guevara Ramos, L. M., G. Gonzales, G. J. Canino, and H. Bird. n.d. "Cross-Cultural Aspects of Psychotic Symptoms in a Hispanic Population." Manuscript.

Guntrip, H. 1969. *Schizoid Phenomena, Object Relations and the Self*. New York: International Universities Press.

Haberman, P. W. 1976. "Psychiatric Symptoms among Puerto Ricans in Puerto Rico and New York City." *Ethnicity* 3:133–144.

Hallowell, A. Irving. 1955. *Culture and Experience*. Philadelphia: University of Pennsylvania Press.

Harwood, Alan. 1977. *Rx: Spiritist as Needed*. New York: John Wiley and Sons.

______. 1988. "A Discussion About Discourse." *Medical Anthropolgy Quarterly* 2(2):99–101.

Heelas, A., and A. Lock, eds. 1981. *Indigenous Psychologies: The Anthropology of the Self*. London: Academic Press. Hidalgo, Hilda, and Elia H. Christensen. 1979. Two

Women: A Story of Success. In Edna Acosta-Belen, ed., *The Puerto Rican Woman*, 142–159. New York: Praeger.

Hill, R., J. M. Stycos, and K. W. Back. 1959. *The Family and Population Control*. Chapel Hill: University of North Carolina Press.

Hillman, James. 1975. *Revisioning Psychology*. New York: Harper and Row.

Hoyt, Michael F. 1980–1981. "Clinical Notes Regarding the Experience of 'Presences' in Mourning." *Omega* 11(2):105–111.

Huberty, C. J. 1975. "Discriminant Analysis." *Review of Educational Research* 45:543–598.

______. 1984. "Issues in the Use and Interpretation of Discriminant Analysis." *Psychological Bulletin* 95:156–171.

Jones, D. 1966. *Sanapia: Comanche Medicine Woman*. New York: Holt, Rinehart and Winston.

Jung, Carl G. 1954. *Collected Works: The Practice of Psychotherapy*. Bollingen Series XX, vol. 16. New York: Pantheon.

______. 1969. *Collected Works*. Vol. 8. 2d ed. Princeton: Bollingen Press.

Kakar, Sudhir. 1982. *Shamans, Mystics, and Doctors*. Boston: Beacon Press.

Kaplan, H. I., and Benjamin J. Saddock, eds. 1985. *Comprehensive Textbook of Psychiatry/IV*. Vol. 1. Baltimore: Williams & Wilkins.

Kardec, Allan. 1883. *Genesis: The Miracles and the Predictions*. Boston: Colby and Rich. Translation of *La Genese, Les Miracles et les Predictions Selon le Spiritisme* (Paris: La Croix, 1868).

______. 1886. *The Spirits' Book*. Boston: Colby and Rich. Translation of *Philosophie Spiritualiste*, 14th ed. (Paris: Didier, 1886).

Katon, Wayne, A. Kleinman, and G. Rosen. 1982. "Depression and Somatization: A Review, Parts 1 and 2." *American Journal of Medicine* 72:127–135, 241–247.

Kendall, L. 1985. *Shamans, Housewives, and Other Restless Spirits: Women in Korean Ritual Life*. Honolulu: University of Hawaii Press.

Kirmayer, L. J. 1984a. "Culture, Affect and Somatization: Part I." *Transcultural Psychiatric Research Review* 21(3):159–188.

______. 1984b. "Culture, Affect and Somatization: Part II." *Transcultural Psychiatric Research Review* 21(4):237–262.

______. 1986. Somatization and the Social Construction of Illness Experience. In S. McHugh and Michael Vallis, eds., *Illness Behavior*. New York: Plenum Publishing Company.

______. 1987. "Languages of Suffering and Healing: Alexthymia as a Social and Cultural Process." *Transcultural Psychiatric Research Review* 24(2):119–136.

Kleinman, Arthur. 1980. *Patients and Healers in the Context of Culture*. Berkeley: University of California Press.

______. 1988. *Rethinking Psychiatry: From Cultural Category to Personal Experience*. New York: Free Press.

Kleinman, Arthur, and L. H. Sung. 1979. "Why do Indigenous Practitioners Successfully Heal?" *Social Science and Medicine* 138:7–26.

Kleinman, Arthur, and Joan Kleinman. 1985. Somatization: The Interconnections in Chinese Society Among Culture, Depressive Experiences and the Meanings of Pain. In A. Kleinman and B. Good, eds., *Culture and Depression*, 429–490. Berkeley: University of California Press.

Kleinman, Arthur, and Byron J. Good, eds. 1985. *Culture and Depression*. Berkeley: University of California Press.

Kohut, Heinz. 1971. *The Analysis of the Self*. New York: International Universities Press.

Konner, Melvin. 1987. *Becoming a Doctor*. New York: Viking Press.

Koss, Joan D. 1965. *Puerto Ricans in Philadelphia: Migration and Accommodation*. Ann Arbor, Mich.: University Microfilms.

______. 1972. Why Cults are Born: The Case of *Espiritismo* in Puerto Rico. In Basil Ince, ed., *Race, Society and Politics in the Caribbean*, 37–54. Rio Piedras, Puerto Rico: Benzal Publishing Company.

______. 1974. "Health and Social Problems in the Community of Bunker, Caguas, Puerto Rico." Report of an investigation submitted to Dr. Jose Nuñez Lopez, Subsecretary for Mental Health, Department of Health of Puerto Rico, August.

______. 1975. "Therapeutic Aspects of Puerto Rican Cult Practices." *Psychiatry* 38:160–171.

______. 1976. "Religion and Science Divinely Related: A Case History of Spiritism in Puerto Rico." *Caribbean Studies* 16:22–43.

______. 1977. "Social Process, Healing and Self-Defeat among Puerto Rican Spiritists." *The American Ethnologist* 4(3):453–469.

______. 1979. Artistic Expression and Creative Process in Caribbean Possession Cult Rituals. In J. Cordwell, ed., *The Visual Arts: Graphic and Plastic*, 373–410. The Hague: Mouton.

______. 1980. "The Therapist-Spiritist Training Project in Puerto Rico: An Experiment to Relate the Traditional Healing System to the Public Health System." *Social Science and Medicine* 14(B):255–266.

______. 1986. "Symbolic Transformations in Traditional Healing Rituals: Perspectives from Analytical Psychology." *Journal of Analytical Psychology* 31:341–355.

______. 1987. "Expectations and Outcomes for Patients Given Mental Health Care or Spiritist Healing in Puerto Rico." *American Journal of Psychiatry* 144:56–61.

La Fontaine, J. 1981. "The Domestication of the Savage Male." *Man* 16:333–349.

Landy, David. 1959. *Tropical Childhood*. Chapel Hill: University of North Carolina Press.

Langs, Robert. 1978. *The Listening Process*. New York: Jason Aronson.

Lavater, L. 1572. *Of Ghosts and Spirits Walking by Night*. London: Watkyns.

Leacock, S., and R. Leacock. 1975. *Spirits of the Deep*. Garden City, N.Y.: Anchor Books.

Lehmann, H. E. 1985. Affective disorders: Clinical Features. In H. Kaplan and B. Saddock, eds., *Comprehensive Textbook of Psychiatry*, vol. 1, 786–811. Baltimore: Williams & Wilkins.

Lehmann, H. E., and R. Cancro. 1985. Schizophrenia: Clinical Features. In H. Kaplan and B. Saddock, eds., *Comprehensive Textbook of Psychiatry*, vol. 1, 680–713. Baltimore: Williams & Wilkins.

LeShan, L. 1974. *The Medium, the Mystic and the Physicist*. New York: Viking Press.

Lewis, Gordon. 1963. *Puerto Rico: Freedom and Power in the Caribbean*. New York: Monthly Review Press.

Lewis, I. M. 1971. *Ecstatic Religion*. Harmonsworth, England: Penguin Books.

Lifton, R. J. 1970. *Boundaries: Psychological Man in Revolution*. New York: Random House.

Littlewood, Ronald, and Maurice Lipsedge. 1987. "The Butterfly and the Serpent: Culture, Psychopathology and Biomedicine." *Culture, Medicine and Psychiatry* 11(3):289–336.

Lopez, S., and Maya Munoz. 1980. *Matrimonio y Divorcio en Puerto Rico desde la Perspectiva de la Mujer*. San Juan, Puerto Rico: University of Puerto Rico.

Lopez Garriga, María Milagros. 1980. Estrategias de Auto-afirmacion en Mujeres Puertorriqueñas. In Edna Acosta-Belen, ed., *La Mujer en la Sociedad Puertorriqueña*. Rio Piedras, Puerto Rico: Ediciones Huracan.

Low, Setha. 1981. "The Meaning of *Nervios*: A Sociocultural Analysis of Symptom Presentation in San Jose, Costa Rica." *Culture, Medicine and Psychiatry* 5(1):25–48.

______. 1985. "Culturally-Interpreted Symptoms or Culture-Bound Syndromes." *Social Science and Medicine* 21:187–196.

Ludwig, Arnold M. 1969. Altered States of Consciousness. In Charles Tart, ed., *Altered States of Consciousness*. New York: John Wiley and Sons.

McClain, C. 1989. *Women as Healers*. New Brunswick and London: Rutgers University Press.

Maldonado Sierra, Eduardo D., R. D. Trent, and F. Fernandez. 1960. "Neuroses and Traditional Family Beliefs in Puerto Rico." *International Journal of Social Psychiatry* 6:237–246.

Mason, J. A. 1960. *Folklore Puertorriqueno: I. Adivinanzas*. San Juan, Puerto Rico: Instituto de Cultura Puertorriqueña.

Mechanic, D. 1972. "Social Psychologic Factors Affecting the Presentation of Bodily Complaints." *New England Journal of Medicine* 286(21):1132–1139.

Medawar, Peter, and Jean S. Medawar. 1977. *The Life Science*. London: Wildwood House.

Mehlman, R. D. 1961. "The Puerto Rican Syndrome." *American Journal of Psychiatry* 118:328–332.

Mirowsky, John M., and Catherine E. Ross. 1984. "Mexican Culture and Its Emotional Contradictions." *Health and Social Behavior* 25:2–13.

Moerman, David E. 1983. Physiology and Symbols: The Anthropological Implications of the Placebo Effect. In L. Romanucci- Ross, D. Moerman, and L. Tancredi, eds., *The Anthropology of Medicine: From Culture to Method*, 156–167. New York: Praeger.

Muñoz Vásquez, Marya. 1979. The Effects of Role Expectations on the Marital Status of Urban Puerto Rican Women. In Edna Acosta-Belen, ed., *The Puerto Rican Woman*, 75–84. New York: Praeger.

______. 1980. Matrimonio y Divorcio en Puerto Rico. In Edna Acosta-Belen, ed., *La Mujer en la Sociedad Puertorriqueña*. Rio Piedras, Puerto Rico: Ediciones Huracan.

Nemiah, J. C. 1985. Anxiety States (Anxiety Neuroses). In H. I. Kaplan and Benjamin J. Saddock, eds., *Comprehensive Textbook of Psychiatry/IV*, vol. 1, 883–894. Baltimore: Williams & Wilkins.

Nichter, M. 1981. "Idioms of Distress." *Culture, Medicine and Psychiatry* 5(4):379–411.

Nieves Falcon, Luis. 1973. *Diagnostico de Puerto Rico*. Rio Piedras, Puerto Rico: Ediciones Edil.

Nuñez Molina, Mario A. 1987. "'Desarrollo del Medium': The Process of Becoming a Healer in Puerto Rican Espiritismo". Ph.D. dis., Graduate School of Education, Harvard University.

Ortner, Sherry. 1974. Is Female to Male as Nature is to Culture? In M. Z. Rosaldo and L. Lamphere, eds., *Woman, Culture, and Society,* 67–87. Stanford: Stanford University Press.

Pandolfi, Mariella. 1990. "Boundaries Inside the Body: Women's Sufferings in Southern Peasant Italy." *Culture, Medicine and Psychiatry* 14(2):255–274.

Pelletier, Kenneth R. 1977. *Mind as Healer, Mind as Slayer* New York: Dell Publishing.

Perls, Frederick S. 1951. *Gestalt Therapy: Excitement and Growth in the Human Personality.* New York: Julian Press.

Personal Narratives Group. 1989. *Interpreting Women's Lives: Feminist Theory and Personal Narratives.* Bloomington, Ind.: Indiana University Press.

Peters, Larry. 1981. *Ecstasy and Healing in Nepal.* Malibu, Calif.: Undena Press.

Peters, Larry, and Douglas Price-Williams. 1980. "Toward an Experiential Analysis of Shamanism." *American Ethnologist* 7:397–413.

Pico, Fernando. 1986. *Historia General de Puerto Rico.* Rio Piedras, Puerto Rico: Ediciones Huracan.

Press, Irwin. 1969. "Urban Illness: Physicians, Curers and Dual Use in Bogota." *Journal of Health and Social Behavior* 10:209–218.

Pressel, Esther. 1977. Negative Spirit Possession in Experienced Brazilian Umbanda Spirit Mediums. In V. Crapanzano and V. Garrison, eds., *Case Studies in Spirit Possession,* 333–364. New York: John Wiley and Sons.

Prince, Raymond. 1976. "Psychotherapy as the Manipulation of Endogenous Healing Mechanisms." *Transcultural Psychiatric Research Review* 13:115–133.

______. 1982. "Shamans and Endorphins: Hypothesis for a Synthesis." *Ethos* 10:409–423.

Richman, Judith. 1984. "Sex Differences in Social Adjustment." *Journal of Nervous and Mental Disease* 172(9):539–544.

Rivera Quintero, Marcia. 1980. Incorporación de las Mujeres al Mercado de Trabajo en el Desarrollo del Capitalismo. In Edna Acosta-Belen, ed., *La Mujer en la Sociedad Puertorriqueña,* 41–66. Rio Piedras, Puerto Rico: Ediciones Huracan.

Rivera Ramos, A. 1985. *La Mujer Puertorriqueña: Investigaciónes Psico-Sociales.* Puerto Rico: Centro Para el Estudio.

Roberts, Robert E. 1981. "Prevalence of Depressive Symptoms Among Mexican Americans." *Journal of Nervous and Mental Disease* 169(4):213–219.

Roberts, R. E., and C. R. Roberts. 1982. "Marriage, Work, and Depressive Symptoms Among Mexican Americans." *Hispanic Journal of Behavioral Sciences* 4(2):199–221.

Rodriguez Cortes, Carmen. 1990. "Social Practices of Ethnic Identity: A Puerto Rican Psycho-Cultural Event." *Journal of Behavioral Sciences.* 12(4):380–396.

Rodriguez Cortes, Sonia. 1986–1987. "Socio-Cultural-Religious Background of Puerto Rican Women." *Homine* 10:277–287.

Rodriguez Ramos, Esther. 1976. *Los Cuentos de Rene Marques.* Rio Piedras, Puerto Rico: Editorial Universitaria (Colección Uprex).

Rogler, Lloyd H., and August B. Hollingshead. 1961. "The Puerto Rican Spiritualist as Psychiatrist." *American Journal of Sociology* 67:17–21.

______. 1965. *Trapped: Families and Schizophrenia.* New York: John Wiley and Sons.

Rothenberg, Albert. 1964. "Puerto Rico and Aggression." *American Journal of Psychiatry* 121:962–970.

Rubel, Arthur, C. W. O'Nell, and R. Collado Ardon. 1984. *Susto*: A Folk Illness. Berkeley: University of California Press.

Rubio, Mario, M. Urdanetta, and J. L. Doyle. 1955."Psychopathologic Reaction Patterns in the Antilles Command." *U.S. Armed Forces Medical Journal* 6:1767–1772.

Ruiz, P., and J. Langrod. 1976. "The Role of Folk Healers in Community Mental Health Services." *Community Mental Health Services* 12:392.

Russell, S.D. 1984. "Curing and Commerce: Changes in an Indigenous Medical Practice in a Highland Philippine Town." *Social Science and Medicine* 18(2):129–137.

Safa, Helen I. 1974. *The Urban Poor of Puerto Rico: A Study in Development and Inequality.* New York: Holt, Rinehart and Winston.

______. 1975. "Class Consciousness Among Working Class Women in Puerto Rico." *Politics and Society* 5:377–394.

Sampson, E. E. 1988. "The Debate on Individualism: Indigenous Psychologies of the Individual and Their Role in Personal and Societal Functioning." *American Psychologist* 43:15–22.

Samuels, Andrew. 1985. "Countertransference, the *Mundus Imaginalis* and a Research Project." *Journal of Analytical Psychology* 30:47–71.

Scarry, E. 1985. *The Body in Pain: The Making and Unmaking of the World.* Oxford: Oxford University Press.

Schapira, Laurie Layton. 1988. *The Cassandra Complex: Living with Disbelief.* Toronto: Inner City Books.

Scheper-Hughes, Nancy, and Margaret M. Lock. 1987. "The Mindful Body: A Prolegomenon to Future Work in Medical Anthropology." *Medical Anthropology Quarterly* 1(1):6–41.

Schieffelin, E. L. 1985. The Cultural Analysis of Depressive Affect: An Example from New Guinea. In A. Kleinman and B. J. Good, eds., *Culture and Depression,* 101–133. Berkeley: University of California Press.

Schwartz-Salant, N. 1982. *Narcissism and Character Formation.* Toronto: Inner City Books.

Singer, Jerome L. 1976. *Daydreaming and Fantasy.* London: George Allen and Unwin.

Snow, L. F. 1977. Popular Medicine in a Black Neighborhood. In E. Spicer, ed., *Ethnic Medicine in the Southwest,* 19–25. Tucson: University of Arizona Press.

SPSS-X, Inc. 1983. *SPSS-X User's Guide.* New York: McGraw-Hill.

Srole, Leo, T. S. Langer, S. T. Michael, M. E. Opler, and T.A.C. Bennie. 1962. *Mental Health in the Metropolis.* New York: McGraw-Hill.

Stoller, Paul. 1984. Eye, Mind and Word in Anthropology. *L'Homme* 24(3–4):91–114.

Thompson, Catherine. 1985. "The Power to Pollute and the Power to Preserve: Perceptions of Female Power in a Hindu Village." *Social Science and Medicine* 21:701–711.

Torres Matrullo, Carmen. 1982. Cognitive Therapy of Depressive Disorders in the Puerto Rican Female. In R. Becerra, M. Karno, and J. Escobar, eds., *Mental Health and Hispanic Americans: Clinical Perspectives.* New York: Greene & Straton.

Tousignant, Michel. 1985. "Pena in the Ecuadorian Sierra: A Psychoanthropological Study of Sadness." *Culture, Medicine and Psychiatry* 9:235–248.

Trautman, E. C. 1961. "The Suicidal Fit." *Archives of General Psychiatry* 5:76–83.

Ulanov, Ann B. 1981. *Receiving Woman: Studies in the Psychology and Theology of the Feminine.* Philadelphia: Westminister Press.

Vasquez-Nuttall, E., I. Romero Garcia, and B. De Leon. 1987. "Sex Roles and Perceptions of Femininity and Masculinity of Hispanic Women." *Psychology of Women Quarterly* 11:409–425.

Vega, Ann Lydia, and Carmen Lugo Filippi. 1981. *Virgenes y Marteres (Cuentos).* Rio Piedras, Puerto Rico: Edit. Antillana.

Vega, William, G. Warhest, J. Buhl-Auth, and K. Meinhardt. 1984. "The Prevalence of Depressive Symptoms Among Mexican Americans and Anglos." *American Journal of Epidemiology* 120:592–607.

Vernon, S. W., and R. E. Roberts. 1982. "Uses of the SADS-RDC in a Tri-Ethnic Community Survey." *Archives of General Psychiatry* 39:47–52.

Wagenheim, Kal. 1970. *Puerto Rico: A Profile.* New York: Praeger.

Wallace, Anthony F. C. 1966. *Religion: An Anthropological View.* New York: Random House.

Warner, Richard. 1976–1977. "The Relationship Between Language and Disease Concepts." *International Journal of Psychiatry in Medicine* 7(1):57–68.

Weissman, Myrna M., and Gerald L. Klerman. 1977. "Sex Differences in the Epidemiology of Depression." *Archives of General Psychiatry* 34:98–111.

Werner, H. 1985. Schizophrenia: Etiology. In H. Kaplan and B. Saddock, eds., *Comprehensive Textbook of Psychiatry,* vol. 1, 650–680. Baltimore: Williams & Wilkins.

Westermeyer, Joseph. 1987a. "Clinical Considerations in Cross- Cultural Diagnosis." *Hospital and Community Psychiatry* 38:160–165.

______. 1987b. "Cultural Factors in the Psychiatric Assessment of Refugees and Others." Manuscript.

Williams, N. A. 1965. "The Magic Helper: A Regressive Variant." *Psychiatry* 28(2):133–144.

Winnicott, David W. 1971. *Playing and Reality.* New York: Basic Books.

Wintrob, Ronald, and Mansell Pattison. 1981. "Possession and Exorcism in Contemporary America." *Journal of Operational Psychiatry* 12:11–20.

Wolf, Katherine. 1952. "Growing Up and Its Price in Three Puerto Rican Subcultures." *Psychiatry* 15:401–433.

Wolff, Toni. 1956. *Structural Forms of the Feminine Psyche.* Monograph privately printed for the Students' Association, C. G. Jung Institute of Zurich.

Index

UNIV DUNELM